Praise for

woman heal thyself

"Jeanne Blum's beautiful book gives women back power and control over their bodies. Healing was always meant to be simple and natural, and she is showing us how."

—LOUISE HAY
AUTHOR, *You Can Heal Your Life*

"With her knowledge of Oriental medicine, the emotions, and addictions, Jeanne Blum is able to take my method one step deeper."

—JOHN LEE
AUTHOR, *The Flying Boy: Healing the Wounded Man* and
Recovery Plain and Simple

"*Woman Heal Thyself* is an important and inspiring practical guide for sustaining emotional and physical health. A must for every woman who cares about herself."

—ANGELES ARRIEN, PH.D., CULTURAL ANTHROPOLOGIST
AUTHOR, *The Four-Fold Way* and *Signs of Life*

"This important and exciting book presents ancient healing methods and the wisdom that Jeanne Blum has accumulated in her years of practice, to help women heal many common health problems."

—SUSAN LARK, M.D.
Women's Health Care & Preventive Medicine

"*Woman Heal Thyself* enables women to better understand their bodies and gives them practical tools to bring themselves into balance. I highly recommend this book."

—CYNTHIA MERVIS WATSON, M.D.
AUTHOR, *Love Potions: A Guide to Aphrodisiacs and Sexual Pleasures*

woman
heal
thyself

*An Ancient Healing System
for Contemporary Women*

Revised Edition

JEANNE ELIZABETH BLUM
M.T., O.M.T.

CHARLES E. TUTTLE CO., INC.
Boston • Rutland, Vermont • Tokyo

First published in 1995 by
CHARLES E. TUTTLE CO., INC.
153 Milk Street, Fifth Floor
Boston, Massachusetts 02109
First paperback edition published in 1996.

Cataloging-in-Publication Data

Blum, Jeanne Elizabeth, 1952
    Woman heal thyself : an ancient healing system
for contemporary women — Rev. ed.
           p. cm.
    Includes bibliographical references and index.
    ISBN 0-8048-3101-7
    1. Women--health and hygiene   2. Alternative medicine
3. Self-care, Health I. Title
RA778.B665 1996   96-8886
613´.04244--dc20   CIP

Illustrations by: Jancis Salerno
Yin Yang symbol: Bill Mason

Warning-Disclaimer

The material in this book should not replace treatment by your doctor. This book presents information and knowledge based on Oriental techniques in use for many years. People's lives have different conditions and stages of growth. The adoption and application of the material offered in this book must be your own responsibility. The author and publisher of this book are not responsible in any manner whatsoever for any injury that may occur through following instructions in this book.

Please Note

Although every effort has been made to credit sources, this book may lack a number of references, including those compiled by my teacher, N. Marchant, whose source list was incomplete. Any authors, living or dead, will happily be credited as soon as they are heard from or located.

Printed in the United States of America
01 00 99 98 97 96   1 3 5 7 9 10 8 6 4 2

This book is dedicated

TO WOMEN EVERYWHERE, and to anyone who has endured pain and ill health while longing for relief and healing.

To those who never cease to ask "why-how-when?" To my husband, Ralph H. Blum, who welcomes those questions—most of the time—and encouraged me to write this book. Without his love and continued support this book might not have been written.

It is also dedicated to all couples who strive to heal their childhood wounds as adults and who have the courage to help each other overcome painful patterns of self- and partner destruction.

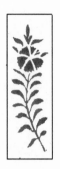

contents

PART SIX
ADDITIONAL TOOLS FOR HEALING

AFTERWORD

APPENDIX A

APPENDIX B

QUICK CHART REFERENCE FOR POINTS

 # acknowledgments

A LIFETIME OF FACES COMES TO MIND AS I PONDER WHERE I have been and those who have helped me along the way. It is my women friends to whom I am most grateful: for their love, support, friendship, and teachings at different times. Sometimes being my friend has been a less-than-easy task, and I thank you all for your perseverance.

Especially my godmother and Aunt Maureen who has always stood by me, no matter what. To Lucille, Jetta, Betty, Lynne, Gerry, Dorothy, Moira, Seonaid, Susie, Jane P., Annie, Kathleen, Debbie, Rovi, Margie, Jaishree, Maria, Barbara, Liz, Joanna, Lydia, Sue, Mary, Beth, Kay, Edythe, Susan, Minette, Dianne, Wende, Meyla, Joan, Margaret, Judy, Connie, Gigi, Jan, Elizabeth, Adelle, Jenny, Jossie, Pat, Kathy, Michelle, Cynthia, Elissa, April, Heather, Iana, Carolyn, Nancy, Caroline, Alta, Joyce, Kirsten and Laurence, Paula and James, Jenny and Bob, my mom and dad, guardian Eric, Bos'n, Mangus, and Curtwist—and the cats who have loved and protected me— thank you all for being in my life. I owe you more than words can ever convey.

Mary Ellen, who read the first two chapters and said "Give me more, this is great!" at a particularly "low" period in my life when her encouragement really helped.

My friend Bronwyn, who helped with my book proposal and whose neat, tidy, wind-chimed house was a delight to enter after leaving a room filled with chapters piled all over my "desk"—the floor.

My Agent, Jane, whose smile is like a welcome hug. Her humor and belief in me and this work gave me the strength to continue after a bad car crash.

Thanks to Jan and her artwork, to Stephan and Hayden, who helped bind the first workbook draft, and especially to Liz, Bill, and Harrison, who taught me assorted computer systems in record time and provided great moral support.

To Becky, who looked after my house and cats in Bermuda while the most crucial part of this writing was done; thank you, from the bottom of my heart, for the peace of mind it afforded me. To Pamela, Elsie, and Shelly, who were always there for me when I picked up the phone and said "Help!"

Deepest thanks to my editor Kathryn, who showed amazing patience and dedication to crafting this book from the original manuscript, and preserving my "voice" throughout her work with my words.

Thanks to my therapists John, Roger, Bruce, Jean, and Jim, my acupuncturist.

Special thanks to Alan and staff, who provided me a quiet work hide-a-way, and to Lynn, who provided a safe place to sleep while I was in New York doing final edits.

Mab Gray, whose wisdom delivered the title of this book.

My husband, Blum, who applied his relentless red pen to this manuscript and encouraged me from the handwritten word to the final days.

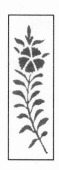

preface

WE HEAR A GREAT DEAL THESE DAYS ABOUT WHAT IT IS TO BE truly feminine, to be a woman "in her power," an earthy, warrior woman, running wild, or breaking the glass ceiling. But what does that really mean if we cannot control the function of our own bodies and we are subject to someone else's idea of politically correct behavior? Actually, it means very little. Words inked and type faced across a page. As women we have come a long way, and yet we still have further to go.

From my twenties onwards I was fully in control of my life, yet in terms of my body, I had been at the mercy of the medical establishment once too often. This does not mean that I had not been helped by traditional Western doctors; I had been helped many times, when my life had been in the balance. What I had grown weary of were the wearing, sometimes debilitating problems that I faced on a monthly basis for which my doctors had no answers. Yes, I could take pain killers, but in the long run, they were hard on my kidneys. And in terms of "edema"—which actually means "a swelling of unknown cause"—well that's all it was; a word. There was no explanation, no insight, no help, and no cure for the painful swelling my legs went through every month prior to my period. I needed to understand why I appeared to be such a gynecological mess. I prayed for help and things began to happen.

About the same time, when I was in my mid-thirties, I had an experience that changed my life. I saw firsthand, to my wonder and awe, the power of healing energy in action. Through the natural healing energy in my hands, I helped a friend heal herself of cervical cancer. I realized then what can happen when we—all of us—are willing and able to heal ourselves. I knew then that I wanted to study healing, but not conventional Western healing.

The question was: Where to begin?

There was so much I did not yet understand about the body. My formal education consisted of boarding school in Scotland, a year of university in San Francisco, and a year at the Academy of Fine Arts in Rome. This was followed by fifteen years in business, during which time I owned and operated a successful cruise company in Bermuda where I was born and raised. I had been married and divorced and was now starting over. What prepared me for the work I now do? My own medical history, the healing gift I'd had since childhood, and a desire to do something worthwhile with my life.

Two days after my decision to leave the business world and start my search for the right kind of training, a brochure from a school 4,000 miles away, across an ocean and a continent, appeared in my mailbox. I had not ordered it and had spoken to no one concerning my strong desire to explore the healing arts. The brochure arrived on a Tuesday and by Thursday I was on a plane headed for the United States.

My studies began with learning massage in order to familiarize myself with the structure and fluid nature of the body. Next, I was drawn to Traditional Oriental Medicine (T.O.M.), which deals specifically with the body's energy flows, flows that the Chinese have been working with for at least 5,000 years. If Oriental medicine is new and unfamiliar to you, think of the flows as being similar to our blood system, only the channels contain energy, the invisible essence and life of our bodies, energy I had been feeling and generating through my hands since I was a child.

The study of Oriental medicine led me to auricular therapy, an acupressure system thousands of years old, through which the entire body—physical and emotional—can be treated by working more than 200 pressure points on the auricle (outer surface) of the ear.

It was during my study of Oriental medicine that I became aware of twenty-four acupressure points that, to my knowledge, have never been fully discussed either in the medical literature or in classical Oriental texts. These points, traditionally known as the Forbidden Pregnancy Points, are so powerful that massaging or needling them on a pregnant woman can seriously disturb—or even terminate—an otherwise normal pregnancy.

In my textbooks, there was sometimes a clear warning about when not to stimulate these points. However, when I asked my teachers how the Forbidden Pregnancy Points could be used in a beneficial way, no one could give me a satisfactory answer.

The Forbidden Points fascinated me; I set out to discover their true nature and usefulness. It was my passionate interest in the Points that ultimately led to healing the numerous gynecological problems that had disrupted my life for twenty-five years—and to the development of the healing system presented in this book: The Forbidden Pregnancy Points System.

Using the Points, I cured myself of premenstrual syndrome (PMS), cramps, an overly-heavy menstrual flow, a class III pap smear situation, and most significantly, endometriosis, a debilitating disease that had plagued me since my early twenties. Encouraged by those results, and with the cooperation of my clients, I began to track other ways in which the Points could be used to bring about healing. In time, I learned to regulate the onset of menstruation and ovulation, and discovered that, by working the Points, the transition into menopause could occur in a more gentle way.

After using this System for many years with my clients, and being asked for information about the Points by a succession of women—including nurses, midwives, therapists and acupuncturists—it became apparent to me that a book like *Woman Heal Thyself* was both timely and necessary.

Where it seemed appropriate, I have shared with you various aspects of my personal life from the early years to the present. So many of us are wounded in one form or another and are survivors. We all have our tales to tell. Opening ourselves to others builds bridges: we form friendships, explore different attitudes, unfamiliar territory, and thereby break down barriers of fear, isolation, and ignorance.

As a survivor of childhood incest, I know only too well the devastating effects abuse can have on one's life and everyday "simple" living, and how, over time, experiences that traumatize us emotionally and spiritually will eventually manifest physically in the body as disease.

By the age of forty, I had survived more major illnesses and accidents than I like to remember. At one point I realized I had undergone twelve operations in a thirteen-year period and had been declared medically dead three times.

Yet these same experiences helped prepare me to become an effective therapist. When I look at a client with empathy and tears in my eyes and say, "I know how you feel," I am listening and speaking from my heart. Having been in a relationship with someone who was addicted and depressed and abusive, I know how difficult and crazy-making that can be. I have been addicted to prescription drugs and nicotine, and I am a survivor of years of sexual abuse. You will never find me in a starched, white lab coat or hear me saying, "Yes, that must have been terrible," while absent-mindedly scribbling notes in the previous patient's file.

Time and again in my life, my choice has been to heal or

die. The demand that I heal myself has given me the tools to help others.

In *Healing and the Mind,* Bill Moyers writes: "Sharing sorrows makes us 'wounded healers,' as C. G. Jung described people whose knowledge of inner healing came from experience with their own wounds. Professionals give advice; pilgrims share wisdom."[1]

I am a combination of professional and pilgrim. In the words of one classical Chinese text, "The doctor's mind should be one with the mind of the patient. The doctor has also to be the patient." With great regularity I have found that the mind is the most important part of the body, since from the mind comes the ability to regulate the energy that travels throughout our bodies, or from one person to another, for healing.

The Forbidden Pregnancy Points System presented in this book is simple, safe, and practical, and can be employed by women everywhere. The basic information about Oriental medicine presented in this book will help you to become familiar with concepts of holistic healing, treating the whole person—the body, the mind, and the spirit—rather than just the few pounds that make up your reproductive organs. Health and spiritual peace come from inside oneself; they are there to seek and find, and cultivate from within.

The success of this System depends on your interest, your needs, and your dedication to yourself. Learn to read your own body, your moods, and your physical symptoms, both healthy and unhealthy. If you purchase this book on a Monday and on Tuesday think to yourself, "I'll just massage a point or two and get rid of PMS . . ." well, quite frankly, you'll be disappointed. There's more to self-awareness and healing than that. Learning to heal rarely takes place over night, and yet you will enjoy the learning process. And what's more, you deserve the time it will take. Keep a personal journal of your healing journey, a place

1. Bill Moyers, *Healing and the Mind* (New York: Doubleday, 1993), p. 319.

where you can record and chart your own physical, mental, and emotional travels over time as you survey your problems, both past and present.

As the principles of Oriental medicine become clear and available to you, you will gain a new understanding of how your body functions, and you will move quickly along the road to freedom from ill health.

It is only in recent years that various aspects of Oriental medicine have begun to take their rightful place alongside allopathic (that is to say, traditional Western) medical techniques and therapies. When the situation warrants it, surgeons in New York, Boston, Dallas, and San Francisco are selectively introducing acupuncture in place of traditional anesthesia, and acupuncture for asthma has been governmentally approved in the United States.

Women have been denied access to these Forbidden Points for over 5,000 years, and yet they are part of a beautiful tradition—a tradition of self-healing and self-regulation—that is our rightful inheritance.

The Forbidden Pregnancy Points System gives women significant control over their bodies, a measure of control we have never had before. Use of the Points involves common sense practices that do not require a diploma or a course of study, for they are part of an available system that any woman can learn, practice, and benefit from alone in her own home.

I am grateful to be able to share with you the Forbidden Pregnancy Points System. You will be surprised and delighted to discover that you can indeed heal yourself.

JEANNE ELIZABETH BLUM
SPRING, 1995

The Yellow Emperor said: "Man has four main arteries and twelve subsidiary vessels."

Ch'i Po answered: "The four main arteries correspond to the four seasons, the twelve vessels correspond to the twelve months, and the twelve months correspond to the twelve pulses.

—FROM THE NEI CHING,
The Yellow Emperor's Classic of Internal Medicine

PART ONE

On the Path
to Healing

I

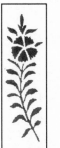

*before
two
clues*

THIS WORK HAD ITS BEGINNINGS MANY YEARS AGO AS A DIRECT result of asking what I thought at the time was a simple question. I had just become aware of information I knew to be critically important to women—information that would allow women to control and manage their bodies, and therefore their lives, from menstruation to menopause and beyond.

This information concerns twenty-four acupressure points. Little research has been done with these twenty-four points. In Oriental medicine they are known traditionally as the "Forbidden Pregnancy Points" and have always been referred to by that term. For over 5,000 years, they have basically been labeled "off limits" during a pregnancy. And while shown on acupuncture charts, these points are never designated or described for their actual positive power and appropriate use. In China, over two thousand years ago, during a time of political repression, the ruler, Ch'in Shih Huang Ti, ordered many books to be heaped on bonfires and destroyed.[1] Perhaps the ancient texts containing this knowledge were committed to those fires.

Writing a complicated Oriental medical text was never my intention. My intention was threefold. One, to help women

1. Richard Wilhelm, translated by C.F. Baynes, *The I Ching* (Princeton: Princeton University Press, 1967), p. xvii.

3

heal themselves using the twenty-four Forbidden Pregnancy Points of Oriental medicine. Two, to bridge the gap between Western medicine—with its heavy reliance on drugs and the scalpel—and Oriental medicine, which, though it is powerful, can seem strange and incongruous to those raised in other cultures. Three, to simplify the knowledge of this complex energy medicine, making it accessible to the everyday Western woman who lives and breathes within a body she may barely understand, a body that may overwhelm and confuse her on a daily, weekly, or monthly basis.

This book was written for women who know nothing about Oriental medicine and even less about the invisible energy that flows, like blood in veins, throughout our bodies—the life force of our very existence.

If just one person who reads this book gains an understanding of why and how we become ill, and the way illness is tied to our emotional state, and how everything in heaven and on earth affects us all so deeply, then I will feel that I have done something worthwhile with my life.

IN FEBRUARY, 1993, a week-long television series on alternative medicine was hosted by Bill Moyers, author of *Healing and the Mind*. It was watched by millions of Americans. In Part I of the series, Moyers went to China to investigate a system of healing that was general knowledge in China more than 5,000 years ago.

We in the West are beginning to recognize that there exists a subtle interconnection of mind, body, and spirit and that this relationship can directly and significantly affect physical healing. Western medicine has been challenged by the ancient Eastern concept of "invisible" energy flowing throughout the body, a network similar to the circulatory system that carries the blood. Oriental medicine is based on these energy flows, which have been known and studied in the East for millennia. In the West—where seeing is believing—we have only recently developed the technology to prove that invisible energy really does flow through the body.

Dr. Kim Bong Han of the University of Pyongang in North Korea discovered that these flows are contained within thin membranes, filled with a colorless fluid. German doctors have found that electricity can be introduced at one point on the flow and it will arrive at the organ with which it is associated. These flows were also noted by Sir Thomas Lewis in 1937, but he did not understand what he had discovered.[2]

More recently, Kirlian photography has captured the healing energy emitted from the hands of healers and practitioners of Oriental medicine who work with this energy—or lack of it. People who are sensitive to energy can actually feel these flows of energy in the body; they can even detect where and when blockages occur. "Energetic body work" is the term used by some therapists for this form of healing.

Acupuncture was originally taught to students of highly evolved meditation, whereby all the pressure points could be mentally activated without touch. Mystics or meditators who have stronger energy than most people can transfer it or increase it in others.[3] Herbs, acupuncture, and laying on of hands all use energy for healing.

This energy, known in Oriental medicine as *ch'i*, is vital to our organs and overall health and must freely circulate in order for the body to be without illness. If the energy pathway becomes blocked, it creates an energetic imbalance in the major organs and, eventually, disease results.

These pathways are usually referred to as "meridians." I like to think of them as "energy flows" just to remind myself

2. Stephen T. Chang, *The Great Tao* (San Francisco: Tao Publishing, 1992), pp. 238, 239.
3. Frena Bloomfield, *The Book of Chinese Beliefs* (New York: Ballantine Books, 1983), p. 110.

that a life force is moving and circulating through our bodies at all times.

Along these energy pathways are located traditional points, precisely defined areas which, when pressed, massaged, or stimulated through acupuncture, increase or decrease the energy along that flow. Once you are familiar with them, these points can be worked—massaged and stimulated—by anyone.

Take a simple example of feeling energy. Perhaps at some time in your life you have experienced the shock of static electricity while standing on a carpet and shaking hands, or pushing an elevator button after being outside in the dead, dry, crisp cold of winter. Not very subtle, but energy all the same. Or perhaps you have had intestinal flu, or food poisoning, and along with the pain or discomfort, you have felt as if you had cold shivers running inside your body. This cold, shivery feeling is energy that has become out of balance. If it was in balance, its presence would not be a nuisance or cause discomfort. Why, if you have intestinal flu, would you have shivers in your arms? Because Large Intestine energy flow begins in the index finger and travels up the arms, and Small Intestine energy flow begins in the little finger and also travels in an upward direction . . . .

The average Westerner connects with energy when he or she puts a plug into a wall socket. That's about as deep or aware as it gets. But we do know what happens when the electricity gets shut off. Well, it's the same with the body.

ONE DAY, DURING my training in acupressure and auricular therapy—a specialized branch of acupressure for treating the entire body from energy points on the ears—our teacher had just finished stressing the power of the Forbidden Pregnancy Points. She stated emphatically that these points should never be massaged, stimulated, worked, or needled during a pregnancy, since a miscarriage would most likely occur in one to three days.

Her eyes surveyed the entire class to make sure this information had registered. Clearly, these points were off limits if someone was pregnant. Or were they? A silence fell over the class as we pondered the significance of her words.

It occurred to me that if these points could have that deep a negative effect on a wanted pregnancy, they must be equally powerful for the specific healing of a woman's body. Oriental medicine is based on the fundamental principle that for everything negative there is a positive for balance.

"So when do we use these points?" I asked.

"That's a very good question," she replied. It was all she said.

At the end of my training, I said goodbye to fellow students, a little sad, knowing I would probably never see them again. When I said goodbye to my teacher, she gazed at me with a strange look in her eyes.

"Find the answer to that question," she said, "and I will sit at your feet as you have sat at mine."

AFTER MY TRAINING, I continued to ask that same question and received similar answers from others in the profession. Many therapists and doctors of Oriental medicine looked at me blankly and asked me what had been my experience. One or two talked about the use of a couple of the points to bring about the delivery of an overdue baby, bring on a late period, or turn the baby at term. Others talked about using these points for nausea or constipation or headaches, but only when a woman was not pregnant.

Yet at mid-month, in a menstrual cycle, someone could be pregnant and not know it. Some women have been three months pregnant and unaware of their condition. My husband's mother, a Hollywood movie star of the silent screen era, was a classic example of this. When she was six months pregnant she actually thought that what she was feeling had to do with something she had eaten! There are even recent cases of women, rushed to the hospital with unknown abdominal pain, who promptly gave birth to full-term babies. So how could you use these points just at "any time" in a monthly cycle for constipation for example, without risk to a wanted, planned pregnancy? Answer is, you couldn't. By the third week of that cycle, you could be pregnant.

From my inquiries within the field of Traditional Oriental Medicine, "forbidden" appeared to be the key word. The subject seemed shrouded in mystery. There were gaps in the knowledge that made no sense to me. There were too many contradictions. It was all too vague. A rule or method that was more than just "forbidden" had to exist.

Too many people knew too little, no one had the answer, and I tired of asking the question, "When do we use them?" On some level I gave up my intensive search, knowing that the answer would come to me when the time was right. Shortly after this change in attitude, and as is often the way with anything mysterious, clues began appearing along the path of discovery.

2

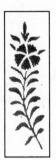 *"so when do we use these points?"*

AFTER I BEGAN MY SEARCH FOR THE ANSWER TO MY question, two incidents provided me with clues to help me understand the mystery of the Forbidden Pregnancy Points.

A male therapist, who was particularly heavy-handed, was giving me a massage one afternoon. He was being rather rough with my ankle areas, where some of the Forbidden Pregnancy Points are located. The massage was extremely painful.

Intuitively, in my gut, I just knew he was doing something wrong. He ignored me when I asked him to stop massaging the area. I finally had to demand that he stop immediately! Three days later my menstrual period began—fifteen days early in a thirty-day cycle. My period never came early. I knew his body-work had brought on my period, and I knew, somehow, that this was important information. I filed the event away in my mind.

The second incident occurred about a month later. While doing volunteer work as an acupressure and auricular therapist at a remote orphanage in Mexico, I came to experience the real power of these Points.

A young woman, four months pregnant, was tumbled in strong surf and began bleeding quite heavily. Her father came looking for the doctor who lived at the orphanage, and finding him away and telephones non-existent, asked for my help. I explained through a translator that I was not a physician, but with the family's permission, I would do what I could to help.

By the time we ran to the beach, his daughter had managed to get herself to their simple brick house. She was indeed bleeding heavily; she was also hysterical. We helped her inside the house, laid her out on her bed, covered her with a blanket to keep her warm, and elevated her legs. It was a small room, probably only nine feet wide and a bit longer. Above the bed there was a picture of the Virgin Mary. The walls were whitewashed, and in the corner stood an old wooden chair with a woven straw seat. A large spider web hung near the ceiling; the floor was clean.

In Traditional Oriental Medicine we begin diagnosis by taking twelve pulses, six in each wrist. Each one of these pulses corresponds to a major organ, such as the liver or kidneys or spleen. Normally a pulse reading will take five or ten minutes, sometimes from twenty minutes to an hour. It is a procedure that connects the practitioner with many aspects of the client's being. While silently monitoring the pulses it is possible to feel, for example, if a person is angry or sad without actually asking any questions about their emotional health. I checked the young woman's pulses to see what state she was in and found the pulse that corresponds to her reproductive organs to be extremely weak and erratic. The sadness in her eyes was almost overwhelming. Four pairs of anxious eyes stared at me with great hope.

Never had I been faced with an emergency situation like this. At a loss about what to do next, I began to pray for help. The first thought that popped into my head while I was praying was: *Use the Forbidden Pregnancy Points.* I told myself that was a stupid idea, since stimulating them would bring about a spontaneous abortion. But at that moment, something strange happened. A sense of great calm came over me. And I thought, "OK, God, if it's these points You want, that's what You'll get !"

When I placed my hands above some of these points on the pregnant woman's lower legs, I could feel a great current of energy rushing from her body. I had never felt energy leaving a person so rapidly, or so strongly. It felt thick, heavy, powerful, almost violent, and I was quite taken aback by it. The same thing happened when I held my hands over her hands: more escaping energy.

Without conscious thought, almost as if I was being guided, moving in slow motion through a very gentle dream, I asked the young woman to clasp her hands, her fingers lightly touching the Forbidden Ho Ku Points on each hand, thereby creating a closed energetic circuit in her upper body.

Next, without touching her, I placed my hands about four inches above her ankles and

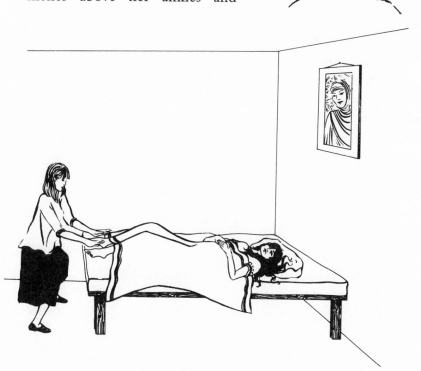

prayed that her energy would stop leaving her body. Somehow, using the healing energy coming from my hands, I "cauterized" or sealed off the energy that was pouring out of these points. Then I consciously pushed healing energy into the Forbidden Pregnancy Points (Spleen 6) in her lower legs. Her crying ceased, her breathing eased, she fell asleep, and within a few minutes, the bleeding stopped.

In the quiet of that simple house, I felt the significance of the healing. Having placed my total trust in a power greater than my own when I was at a loss for direction or procedure, I had been given the answer to my original question: "When do we use these points?"

Suddenly I simply knew, as if a lightbulb had turned on inside my head, that the points should be stimulated and worked (needled or massaged) when we know we are *not* pregnant—when we menstruate—and worked until the pain in the points is diminished.

Ironically, in daring to break the cardinal rule on the use of these points, a baby had been saved. I also realized, in the flood of information that poured into, or out of my brain, that the Forbidden Pregnancy Points can help women to heal menstrual problems and regulate their entire cycle. I knew by using all the points, a healing system could be developed.

3

guinea pig phase

I WAS ON THE PATH TO PROVING WHAT I KNEW DEEP INSIDE TO be true. Using myself as a guinea pig, some wonderful changes happened.

My own history was one of terrible pre-menstrual syndrome (PMS): headaches, bloating, weight gain, irritability, breast tenderness and enlargement, unquenchable thirst, sugar cravings. Sometimes I would burst into tears for little or no reason during the entire week before my period was due.

When my period actually began, the bleeding was extremely heavy, with cramps so severe that, as a teenager, I would regularly black out from pain. During menstruation, I was plagued by alternating constipation and diarrhea, nausea, vomiting, fever, pain and numbness down my right leg, and water retention. I also had endometriosis—which accounts for 20 to 50 percent of infertility in women today. Endometriosis is a condition in which the endometrial cells lining the womb go "wild" and can attach themselves outside the womb onto the cervix, ovaries, fallopian tubes, or within the peritoneal cavity.

Over a four-year span, beginning at the age of twenty-nine, I had a "chocolate cyst," had my right ovary and fallopian tube removed, a cyst removed from the surface of my left ovary, endometrial cells cauterized on the cervix, and erosion of the cervix repaired. During this same time period, one doctor said that the terrible pain in my right leg was only in my mind. Eventually, as I learned more about the points, I discovered that the problem was caused by a blockage in the Spleen energy flow attempting to travel up my leg.

So, in the guinea pig stage, I began to experiment with myself, going from using the most powerful of the points to those that had a much more subtle effect, and served generally to balance the body's energy flow. Being sensitive to my own energy flows, I became aware of where the blocks were, where there was no energy at all, or where there was too much energy. When I massaged the points during my periods for three consecutive cycles, each of those periods was remarkably different. By the fourth month, PMS had vanished.

The first difference I noticed was that during my thirty-day cycle, I no longer had water retention in my legs. This problem had bothered me terribly, especially when I was living in a hot, humid climate. Also, my legs had always swollen during air flights, and this no longer happened. The premenstrual abdominal bloating, breast tenderness and enlargement, constant thirst and sugar cravings, teary outbursts, and crabbiness during the week preceding my period, all vanished one by one. When my period did begin, the bleeding was heavy for three days, finished by the fourth day; there was no uterine cramping, no pain down my leg, and bowel problems disappeared. I stopped throwing up throughout the day, and there was no menstrual odor.

The problems that had plagued me since the onset of menstruation at age twelve gradually disappeared to the point where I would wake up, trundle off to the bathroom, and simply discover that I was bleeding. My period became so gentle and nonintrusive to my daily life that I scarcely knew I had it. I had finally achieved a life without pain-killers. Later, I discovered that my endometriosis was gone.

But why so much trouble with this area of my body? And

why had I suffered from kidney disease—pyelonephritis and nephritis—and bladder infections since childhood? Looking back now, five years into my own recovery and examination of my entire medical history, the answer is simple. From the time I was in the cradle until eleven years of age, I was sexually abused many times a week. My first conscious thought while I stared at the ceiling was, "If I could sit up there I could watch over myself. No one could hurt me." The memory of the wish remained, but the reason behind it vanished.

In order to survive, I taught myself—as so many other abused children have done—to "leave" my body at night. On some level I, my Soul, was not there, only my body suffered the abuse.

As I grew up, I lost all memory of the abuse, blocking it out for thirty-eight years until the night my husband rolled over on me as I slept. That night, face down in the mattress I began to suffocate, and with the shock of that physical suffocation, came the memory of a pillow being placed over my face to muffle my cries of protest while I was a baby in the cradle. And I mean baby in the cradle. The abuse started when I was less than ten months old.

When my abuser died I had the "privilege" of sorting through his bank safe deposit box collection of baby porno pictures. Even then, I did not connect the baby in the photos to me; they were shocking photos but it was just "a baby." Now, having remembered my abuse, I knew why I had learned to leave my body at night.

My abuse was so bad, so deeply buried, that it actually took the physical action of suffocation to activate the memories. I probably would have spent years in a therapist's office talking about my idyllic childhood, and wondering why I had so much trouble coping with life, people, my ovaries, and the price of eggs.

The sexual abuse caused trauma that remained in the physical body's "memory," and disease resulted in my pelvic area. Not only sexual abuse, but all childhood emotional wounds, physical and emotional rape, are stored in body memory in this area. And if not dealt with, these body memories will physically manifest into illness and eventually disease.

4

a
birthday
lesson

SOME YEARS AGO, I HAD QUITE A MEMORABLE BIRTHDAY. I WAS taught another important aspect of Traditional Oriental Medicine, and was provided with a strong confirmation of the power of the Forbidden Pregnancy Points.

My boyfriend was halfway across the world on business and, with a seventeen-hour time difference, it was my time to begin waking and his time to begin sleeping. Thoughts of sleeping were not on his mind. He was in bed with an old lover.

I woke up on the floor; I was actually thrown out of bed. My gut reaction, "sick feeling" radar was switched on. I picked up the telephone, got him on the line and demanded to know, what was he doing?! Seeing as I was a raving banshee, he did not bother to deny anything.

So psychically joined to my partner was I, that my Soul knew when he was being unfaithful, or perhaps his own Soul was so horrified at his behavior that it called out to me from the other side of the world.

Shaken and feeling peculiar, I realized that I was bleeding. I had also been feeling a bit odd in recent mornings—dizzy, sensitive to smells, craving Big Macs (which was not like me)— but I had been so busy plastering, painting, and wallpapering our apartment that my body had been at the bottom of my "focus" list. The only thing I was in touch with was my paint-brush.

I spent the morning of my birthday in writing class, mas-saging my Forbidden Pregnancy Points on and off between paragraphs. Class was held in the comfort of the teacher's home and I was sitting in a big, roomy, comfortable arm chair with my legs uncrossed—tucked up in front of me—which made it con-venient for reaching into my lap area to press points on my feet and legs, as well as the Ho Ku points between my thumb and forefinger.

That night, a highly intuitive friend came over for my party, walked in the door and said, "Hello darling—you're preg-nant. There is child energy around you! Happy birthday."

I looked at her in horror, the memory of all the odd feel-ings I'd had of late finally sinking in. "Oh Edythe," I replied, "I've been working my Forbidden Pregnancy Points all day! I started to bleed and thought it was an early period because of the emotional stuff I was picking up."

As calmly as possible, I called an acupuncturist, who was also coming for dinner, and asked her to get there as soon as she could. In my heart I knew, yet refused to accept, that I had helped myself lose the child I so desperately wanted to have before my biological clock ran down. I stayed in bed for three days, drinking Chinese herbal tea, working my anti-miscarriage points until I wept. But it was of no use.

Again, the truth of something I had learned from my teacher, and had been dutifully passing on to my clients, was powerfully demonstrated to me. According to Oriental thought, a woman physically processes the emotional garbage for the man, or men, with whom she partners sexually. In the Oriental view, when a woman has her period, she is also clear-ing out her partner's emotional turmoil or pain or grief or fear or whatever he has been going through that month.

What was your period like this month? Did you have more cramping? Heavier flow than normal? Has your partner been having a hard time? According to the Oriental way of thinking—that women physically process the emotions of their male partners—you are most likely going to experience difficult menstrual periods, and probably a great deal of pain or cramping from processing and discharging *his* emotional baggage.

So, if you are following the System of monthly points massage as outlined in this book, and are still having problems when you bleed, then please take a very serious look at the emotional and spiritual health of your partner. Especially if you have cleared up all your PMS symptoms. You might want to reevaluate your partnership, however painful that may be.

There is another aspect to this processing of emotional garbage. I have heard stories of women who had terrible difficulties with their periods when their children were going through rough times, and of a woman who was very close to her sister and developed menstrual problems during the sister's divorce.

It must also be pointed out that, aside from the possibility that your partner, or a close family member, may be having emotional difficulties, you could have a serious physical condition that needs to be attended to by a physician. Persistent pain, discomfort, odd physical sensations, or changes in your body should never be ignored.

My own traumatic birthday experience also reemphasized the importance of working the points *only* when you know you have your period, and *not* if you get breakthrough bleeding at any other time of the monthly cycle. Do not assume, as I did, that your normal menses simply arrived a few days early.

PART TWO

Understanding the Basics of Chinese Medicine

5

ancient female teachers

THE HISTORY OF TRADITIONAL ORIENTAL MEDICAL KNOWL-
edge is steeped in folklore that dates back well over 5,000 years.
This knowledge is said to have come from women, including
three immortal sisters, known as the Dark Girl, the Plain Girl,
and the Elected Girl.

This fact—that women were master teachers—is rarely
mentioned in books on Oriental medicine, although it is an
integral part of Taoist tradition. Taoism (pronounced *dow*-ism)
is an ancient Chinese philosophy that advocates, among other
things, simplicity, selflessness, and teaches how to physically love
in an appropriate manner, thereby creating complete harmony
between man and woman. "Tao" literally translates as "the way
the universe works." [1]

In ancient China, men and women clearly understood that
for there to be harmony between the sexes, there had to be sat-
isfaction for both partners in their lovemaking. As a result, beautiful rituals came into the art of loving. One ancient text lists
thirty different positions for lovemaking, the positions having
names like Loving Swallows, Flying White Tiger, Leaping Wild

1. R. L. Wing, *The Tao of Power*, first edition (New York, Doubleday: 1986), p.9.

Horses, Turning Dragon or the somewhat whimsical, Cat and Mouse Share a Hole.[2]

A man understood that he had to satisfy his woman completely, as well as himself, for this harmony to exist. Lovemaking in ancient China took hours; it was never hurried, because each stage of sexual arousal was known to produce bodily secretions in the woman, the release of which were of great benefit to both partners.

The ancients gave these fluids lovely names, and believed that *Jade Spring* came from the saliva as a result of deep erotic kissing; kissing and sucking the nipples produced sweet tasting *White Snow*. The release of this fluid from the nipples has nothing to do with childbearing, and the energetic quality of the fluid is actually better if the woman hasn't borne a child, and the fluid is not breast milk or colostrum. When this fluid is secreted it is said to help regulate the periods, actually relieve menstrual cramps, and improve blood circulation in the woman. The third fluid is *Moon Flower* from the Palace of Yin (womb) when orgasm occurs. It was well-known that these secretions were beneficial to the male, enhancing his own store of feminine energy.

Also, when *Moon Flower* is absorbed by the male through his mouth and tongue during oral sex, the pineal and pituitary glands are activated in the male and help to focus and open the feminine, intuitive part of his mind. From this part of the brain, known as the mind's eye or the Third Eye, total conscious, clear thinking occurs. In turn, the man's energy, without ejaculation, was considered to be beneficial to his woman, and would keep her free from all illness. The purpose of non-ejaculation was to spare the woman being bombarded regularly with the male energy essence, which when absorbed by the woman could cause imbalance within her female system.

The ancients understood that harmony was possible only

2. Jolan Chang, *The Tao of Love and Sex* (New York: Viking Penguin, 1977).

when love and sex combined. Sex for its own sake was a point-less waste of energy. Masturbation was not encouraged in the male because of the loss of his vital male essence, which then could lead to imbalance within his body. However, masturbation was considered beneficial to women, who have a naturally unlimited supply of the female Yin essence, which is replenished on a monthly basis. Release of the female essence through self-gratification is actually nourishing to a woman's physical body and spirit. Anal sex was frowned upon because—especially when it led to ejaculation—it reverses the energy flow entirely, stretches and weakens the anal sphincter muscle, and causes imbalance in the large intestine and the entire digestive tract, which may eventually result in candida or even rectal cancer.

Taoism also teaches that "the feminine element in human life is strongly emphasized, and mythically and historically counts very many women among its greatest teachers."[3]

The Three Immortal Sisters were known by various love-ly names: The Dark Girl (Hsuan-Nu), as "The Peach of Immortality;" The Elected Girl (Ts'ai-Nu), as "The Goddess of Many Colors;" and The Plain Girl (Su-Nu), as "The Queen of the White River" or "Goddess of the Shell."

The sisters taught The Yellow Emperor (Huang-Ti, "The Son of Heaven") everything he wanted to know about any-thing, from sexual secrets to military maneuvers. The compass was invented for him during a time of war by the Queen of the Wind, another immortal female. It was his practice of the Tao of Sex, as taught to him by Su-Nu and her sisters, that allowed Huang-Ti to reign for one hundred years (from 2698 to 2598 B.C.).[4] Their conversations on the art of love are still informative:

> *Huang-Ti*: I am weary and in disharmony. I am sad and appre-hensive. What shall I do about this?

3. Thomas Cleary, *Immortal Sisters,* first edition (Boston: Shambhala, 1989), p.1
4. Chang, *The Tao of Love and Sex*

Su-Nu: All debility of man must be attributed to the faulty ways of loving. Woman is stronger in sex and constitution than man, as water (Yin) is stronger than fire (Yang). Those who know the Tao of Loving are like good cooks who know how to blend the five flavors into a tasty dish. Those who know the Tao of Loving and harmonize the Yin (female) and the Yang (male) are able to blend the five joys into a healthy pleasure; those who do not know the Tao of Loving will die before their time, without ever really having enjoyed the pleasure of loving. Is this not what your Majesty should be looking into?

Hsuan-Nu: In our universe all lives are created through the harmony of Yin and Yang. When Yang has the harmony of Yin all his problems will be solved and when Yin has the harmony of Yang all obstacles in her way will vanish. One Yin and one Yang must constantly assist one another. And thus the man will feel firm and strong. The woman will be ready to receive him into her. The two will thus be in communion and their secretions will nurture each other.[5]

Huang-Ti advised the practice of preventive medicine and the monitoring of the pulses. He believed that seven emotions, when either excessive or insufficient, can affect the body adversely. These emotions are pensiveness, sadness, grief, fear, fright, anger, and joy.[6] It is Huang Ti, the Yellow Emperor, an ancient spiritual adept, who is credited with writing *The Yellow Emperor's Classic of Internal Medicine,* or the *Huang Ti Nei Ching,* from which all medical practice evolved. It is the Bible of Chinese medicine.

The Yellow Emperor's mother was Fu Bao, wife of a tribal chief. His own conception had spiritual associations—it is said that his mother felt energy impregnate her from a star orbiting the Big Dipper. From time to time, he would pray to the Mystical Female from the Big Dipper who sent him his spiritual teachers. He spent nearly twenty years studying Taoist

5. Chang, *The Tao of Love and Sex*, pages 30 and 32. Reprinted by permission.
6. R. L. Wing, *The Tao of Power,* hexagram number 12, First edition, 1986.

spiritual practices and medicine. "Yellow" referred to the centeredness of his energy. It is written that he eventually flew away on a Yellow Dragon when he departed this world.

Lao-tzu, the Old Master, who reputedly lived in the sixth century B.C. and wrote the Taoist classic book *The Way and Its Power* (*Tao-te Ching*, pronounced dow-der-jing) also had a female teacher, the Celestial Mother of Violet Light.[7]

Taoist practice existed in ancient antiquity, long before Lao-tzu or Huang-Ti wrote about it. In that time of legends, again it was a woman who gave the Chinese back their sanity and balance when they were about to destroy themselves and were no longer at one with nature. This "female tribal leader of high antiquity is said to have patched the sky with five-colored stones and given her people the doctrine of the five forces, or five elements,"[8] which is the basis for Oriental medical thought. It was rather like Moses receiving the clay tablets when he was on the mountain with God.

IN ORDER TO place the Forbidden Pregnancy Points in perspective, I must first introduce you to the system to which they belong—Traditional Oriental Medicine. In considering this method of viewing the body and its ills, we will also look at the emotions and their dysfunction.

The Oriental method of medicine is complex; the basics, however, are simple. My intention from the start of writing this book was never to go into the great details of this system or to bog the novice down with long Chinese terms and names. I aim, rather, to break down the information as clearly as possible so that you will have a fundamental understanding of how, without apparent thought, we create illness and disease within our bodies, do it repeatedly, and then wonder how "it" happened . . . again.

7. *Immortal Sisters*, p.63.
8. *Immortal Sisters*, p. 2.

The essence of this system of health maintenance begins with Yin Yang Theory and Five Element Theory. In ancient China people went to doctors, not necessarily because they were sick, but rather to maintain good health. A general rule of thumb was that "The Great Healer can treat the problem before the disease manifests, the medium healer treats the disease after it has appeared."[9] The ancient Chinese understood that spirit, mind, and emotion contributed to physical well-being. Ideally, we could all live in a pure state—proper diet, thoughts, exercise, breathing, sleep, and sexual practice—a state of balance.

The Taoist sage Chuang-tzu, who died around 300 B.C., characterized people of the times who were healthy in mind and body in this manner:

> They did not forget where they had come from, they did not care about where they should pass to; readily they accepted what was alloted to them, peacefully they awaited their decease. It is this that is called "not resisting the Tao [Divine Absolulte]."[10]

Once you understand how Five Element and Yin Yang thought works, I doubt that you will ever cry again, without thinking "Lung" or smile again without thinking "Heart." You will be able to understand the root cause of dis-ease—the body is no longer at ease—and consequently help yourself and those whom you love, to stay healthy.

This book is intended as a map or series of maps. One map will show the routes of energy moving between the points. Another map will chart the path taken by repressed grief, fear, and anger through the territory of the body as a whole and show how the physical organs of the lungs, kidneys, and liver correlate with these emotions as they are processed and eliminated. We will look at how mind, emotion, and spirit affect the

9. Kiiko Matsumoto and Stephen Birch, *Five Elements and Ten Stems*, First edition (Brookline, MA: Paradigm Publications, 1983) p. 63.
10. *Encyclopedia Britannica*, vol. 17, p. 437, 1991.

physical body. Road maps are usually quite easy to read; they are also essential if you want to go anywhere for the first time.

The places on your body that you will eventually visit are listed on many acupuncture reference guides as XP8, XP3, XP4, and XP1. The "XP" stands for "Forbidden Pregnancy" and the number stands for the month during pregnancy from which time onward the point must not be worked. These points also have magical names: Blazing Valley, Palace of Weariness, Heavenly Well, and Joining the Valleys.

When you are ready to learn about this energy system, you will find the theory simply explained in Part Two of this book, and specific instructions for healing in Part Three.

Here then is the essential and simple, bonded to the mysterious. And the reward? A gift of healing to women of all ages, a gift 5,000 years overdue.

6

the yin and yang of all things

THE ANCIENT CHINESE PHILOSOPHERS BELIEVED THAT THE material universe was formed when the Creator achieved self-awareness. In this self-awareness, the Creator knew that he was omnipotent and could create anything that he desired. After the desire and the thought form faded, the energy of that thought turned into matter.[1]

The ancient Chinese believed that everything in the universe was made up of negative and positive flowing energy, that opposites attract, thus creating balance. Balance resulted in harmony.

Within each negative dwelt a positive and within each positive there could be found a negative. When the ancients spoke of negative and positive they were not talking about good and bad. They were referring to the whole cycle of life; active and passive, light and dark, day and night, birth and death, growth and decay, masculine and feminine.

They called this energy Yin (negative) and Yang (positive). The universe, complete in its duality, was ever-changing, merg-

1.Stephen T. Chang, *The Great Tao*, Fourth edition (San Francisco: Tao Publishing, 1992), p.19.

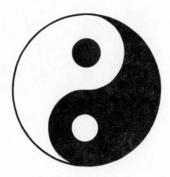

Yin Yang symbol representing the harmony and balance of opposites.

ing in and out of itself as critical mass peaks, with each depen-
dent on the other for balance and wholeness.

The concept of Yin and Yang, or "opposing principles,"
was established by the emperor Shen Nong in 3494 B.C. During this period, through careful observation of everyday life,
"the art of medicine" was born, according to the great Han
dynasty (202 B.C. to 220 A.D.) historian, Sima Qian. This "careful observation of life" is described in one legend, which tells
of a farmer who, upon finding a snake near his house, beat the
snake with a hoe and left it for dead. A few days later, the snake
again appeared, and once more the farmer beat it until it bled.
The impervious reptile slithered off into the grass and began to
eat a particular clump of weeds. By the next morning, the
snake's wounds were healed and the snake was back to slither-
ing about on snake business. And so *San qi* was discovered, the
main ingredient of the remedy *Yunnan bai yao*, a white powder
that stops internal and external bleeding.

Chinese historians credit the development of herbal medicine to Shen Nong, who tested the medicinal effects of hundreds of plants, animals, insects, and seashell extracts, creating
prescriptions that are still in use today in modern China.[2]

Yin and Yang theory preceded Five Element thought, the

2. Daniel P. Reid, *Chinese Herbal Medicine* (Boston: Shambhala Publications, 1993), p.
10.

latter being the theoretical basis for Traditional Oriental Medicine. The ancients knew that within Yang there was Yin and within Yin there was Yang. Yang is male and Yin is female. For example, daytime and sunlight are considered to be Yang, night and darkness are Yin. However, in the late afternoon, when it begins to get dark, still there is light. Because of the darkness, this part of the day—dusk—would be said to be the Yin part of day (Yang). Just before dawn, when the sun is rising, when the sky is still dark, would be the Yang part of night (Yin).

Yin was considered to be more durable than Yang. The ancients observed this in water (Yin), which could erode rock (Yang) over time, and that a fire (Yang) also could be put out by water. Even though fire can boil water away to "nothing," that "nothing" does in fact rise as steam, which is moisture in the air.

These principles also apply to humankind. Within each sex are found aspects of the opposite sex for balance. The gentle, caring, protective aspects of a man's nature are said to be his Yin qualities. The ability of a woman to make firm decisions and take control of situations is regarded as a Yang quality.

Each body organ is said to be masculine or feminine; for example the kidney is Yin and the bladder Yang. The right side of the body is the Yang (male) side, the left side, the Yin (female) side. Does a woman injure herself on the left side more than on the right side, when denying her feminine nature, her feelings, and emotions in some way? Does one side of the body, I wonder, collect more breast lumps than the other?

A woman I met recently has a tragic history, yet she sees her life as a total triumph over everything thrown in her path. One day her ex-husband kidnapped her young children. She never saw them again. Understandably devastated by this terrible emotional trauma, like many people she internalized her loss as she tried to get on with her life. Her sense of self-worth was hardest hit, for she defined herself by her role as a wife and a mother. Traditional Oriental Medicine would say that, on an emotional and subconscious level, she "told" herself she no longer had physical reasons to be a woman. She had no need of breasts to nourish her missing children; without a husband, no need for a womb to make other children. The depth of her ever-present emotional anguish was so great that it manifested throughout her body as disease as it ravaged its way "free." The disease it manifested was cancer. She eventually underwent a hysterectomy and double mastectomy.

Having come to terms with cancer, through traditional Western medicine as well as non-traditional medicine and meditation, she was inspired to change professions in mid-life. She is now a wonderful hands-on healer.

She also learned something very important about what it means to be "female." Despite her operations, she still has an extremely sensual and feminine essence. She has never lost her feminine energy and is every bit "woman"—more so in many ways than some I know who are physically intact. *The feminine energy resides within*; the female essence has nothing to do with parts and appendages.

When I was no longer being sexually abused, the abuse turned into the emotional, verbal type. As a teenager my build was slim with small breasts, and I was encouraged to "eat porridge to put meat on those ribs." This was very hurtful to me because I liked being slim. After some years of verbal and emotional abuse, I began to think that I was deformed and ugly and hated my breasts because they were small. I began hiding in baggy clothes to cover my shamefully imperfect body.

At twenty-three, I went to my gynecologist for a routine visit. He discovered that I had developed lumps in my left breast. A mammogram and thermogram both came back with positive results.

My doctor was not knife-happy. He looked at me intently and said "I want you to come back in a month for another set of tests before we consider doing anything else. I also want you to think about what might have caused this condition. You are very young to have this happen to you."

I returned home and reluctantly told my first husband the bad news. Thrown in was the hopeless comment, "My breasts are so small and ugly, who'll notice anyway if they're gone...?" I turned to hide my face in shame. He grabbed me by the arm, and whirled me around. Furious at my comment, he led me into the bathroom and stood me before the mirror, telling me to "Stay there until you can see how beautiful you are." It was just what the universe ordered. His point hit home. Although his words were roughly delivered, somehow the shock of that unusually forceful sentence broke through the barriers erected from years of verbal abuse, and all the inappropriate comments about my breasts. A true case of Yin and Yang in action. For everything negative there is a positive.

For a long time I stayed there, staring in the mirror at the reflection of my small breasts. It was winter and the apartment was cold, but it didn't seem to matter. As I looked at myself, years of unkind words came back to me. I felt sorry for my abuser, and wondered who had abused him as a child. And I cried for both of us. For the first time in my life I realized that I was not at all deformed or ugly but really quite pretty, and I smiled. With those tears and that smile came healing. The reflection in the mirror became my friend, and I began to have pleasant thoughts about my body, probably for the first time.

A month later I returned to see my doctor. The lumps no longer registered "positive." In fact, there was only one lump and it was very, very tiny. My doctor was not surprised when I shared my story with him. He was the first doctor of traditional Western medicine who told me that thought and feeling had a great deal to do with the body's health. That was back in 1974. Hopefully things will continue to improve within conventional medicine as the gap between East and West continues to close.

Both my husband and my doctor taught me something; they taught me a lesson about right thinking. Right thinking about me, how I had been trained to look at myself and my body. The time had come to view myself with gentler and kinder eyes. The lesson had arrived none too soon.

Here then is a list of Yin and Yang associations and qualities, things that are considered to be female or male in their energetic make up. Learn to think in terms of balance.

YANG	YIN
Male	Female
Sun	Moon
Heaven	Earth
Full Moon	New Moon
Light	Dark
Hot, warm	Cold, cool
Dry	Wet
Dryness	Dampness
Positive	Negative
Energy	Matter
Ascending	Descending
Full	Empty
Change	Constancy
Physical reality	Spiritual reality
Spring, Summer	Fall, Winter
Fire	Water
High	Low
Noble	Common
Left Brain	Right Brain
Transforming	Forming
Hyperactive	Lethargic
Conscious	Subconscious
Acute disease	Chronic disease

YANG	YIN
Excess	Deficient
Virtue	Vice
Joy	Sadness
Order	Confusion
Wealth	Poverty
Rising	Falling
Thoughts	Feelings
Mental function	Emotional function
Active	Passive
Assertive	Receptive
Extroverted	Introverted
Analytical	Intuitive
Rigid	Flaccid
Sympathetic	Parasympathetic
Exterior	Interior
Back	Front
Above	Below
Superficial	Deep
Skin	Bones
Ch'i	Blood
Bright colors	Pastel colors
Red, orange, yellow	Blue, green, purple
Salty, bitter, spicy	Sweet, sour, bland
Grain, animal	Fruit, vegetable
Stomach	Spleen
Large Intestine	Lung
Bladder	Kidney
Gallbladder	Liver
Small Intestine	Heart
Triple Warmer	Pericardium
Governing Vessel	Conception Vessel

Looking at this list, are you *constant* in your relationships, or *changeable*? What effect must that have on your partner? Are your actions ruled by your *conscious* or your *subconscious*? If you have an illness, is it *acute* or *chronic*? Is your life *orderly* or full of *confusion*, resulting in general *chaos*? Do you wear *bright* colors or *pastel* colors? What about the foods you prefer, *salty* or *sweet*?

When you tally up your traits, are you primarily Yin? Or Yang?

These Yin and Yang associations will help you to observe the world and yourself, give you insights into other people, and enable you to look with eyes that see more than they ever saw before.

7

understanding the flow of energy

THERE ARE TWELVE PRIMARY CHANNELS OR MERIDIANS
with energy moving, or flowing, through them—like a
river—in different parts of the body. Eleven of those flows
belong to specific organs and are named for them: Spleen/Pancreas, Stomach, Lung, Large Intestine, Kidney, Bladder, Liver,
Gallbladder, Heart, Small Intestine, and Pericardium (the sack in
which the heart sits). The twelfth flow is known as Triple
Warmer, a flow that regulates all the organs' energies.

There are also eight miscellaneous flows of energy. However, out of those eight, we will be looking at only two, the
Governing Vessel and Conception Vessel. Three-hundred-sixty-five connecting channels[1] also exist; for our purposes it is
unnecessary to go into those flows here—the basics are quite
sufficient!

The flows behave in a way similar to a river; they have a
beginning and an end. The energy is weaker at the beginning
of the flow than it is at the end. They "collect" in energy
strength as they move along. There are points along the flows
where one flow connects with another, called, reasonably

1. John O'Connor and Dan Bensky, Shanghai College of Traditional Medicine,
Acupuncture: A Comprehensive Text, Sixth edition (Seattle: Eastland Press, 1988), p.82.

enough, Connecting Points. Because they connect, they can be used to treat one another. Again, like a river, the flows can be regulated in certain places—Control Points—or they have areas where the energy pools or collects—Source Points—and where the energy is very strong. There are places on the river where the flow can be increased—Tonification Points—if there is too little energy, or decreased—Sedation Points—if there is too much energy. Also like a river, there are places where the river meets a large sea—Accumulation Points; in the case of our bodies, it is where energy actually meets blood. Finally, there are areas of one river that will affect another river—Horary Points—by helping energy to flow in or flow out of the other.

Understanding how the flows interact will be important when you begin to use the Forbidden Pregnancy Points System outlined in Part Three. In chapter 25, I will go into greater depth on how to regulate, control, tonify, and sedate the points you will be working with. At this stage, it is only necessary to understand the nature of the flows, to be aware that energy is constantly moving within your body.

Each one of the twelve primary flows has a pulse—located as six pulses in each of the two wrists—which can be felt to determine the health and state of that flow. When an Oriental medical practitioner or therapist takes your pulse, she or he is feeling twelve pulses, not just one as in Western medicine. Some pulse readings have been known to take over an hour. As you might imagine, it can take many years of study just to learn to accurately read these subtle pulses.

The entire flow of organ-associated vital energy moves throughout the body from one organ to the next, over every twenty-four-hour time period. Each organ flow has its own peak two-hour time slot when the energy is at its strongest. The peak hour for the stomach energy flow, for example, is between 7-9 A.M., a good time to eat breakfast.

Pages 42 through 55 present diagrams of the twelve primary flows in the body, as well as the two additional flows, that we will be looking at.

Each diagram has numerals along the flow to indicate the acupressure point used to "work" energy along the flow. The encircled numerals indicate the twenty-four Forbidden Pregnancy Points. We will look specifically at these points in Part Three.

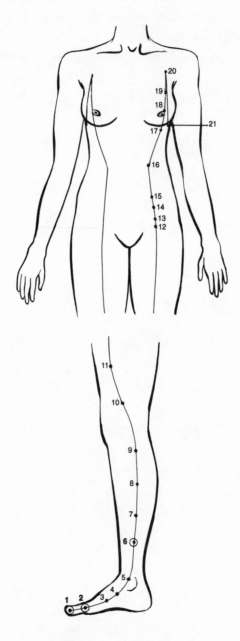

SPLEEN ENERGY FLOW

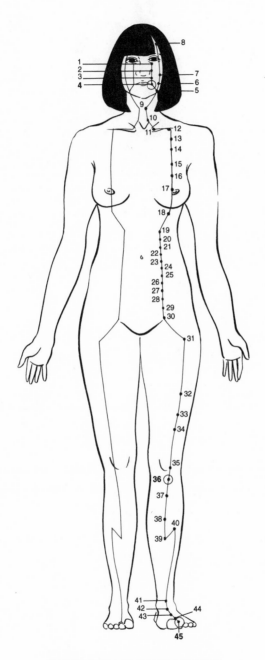

STOMACH ENERGY FLOW

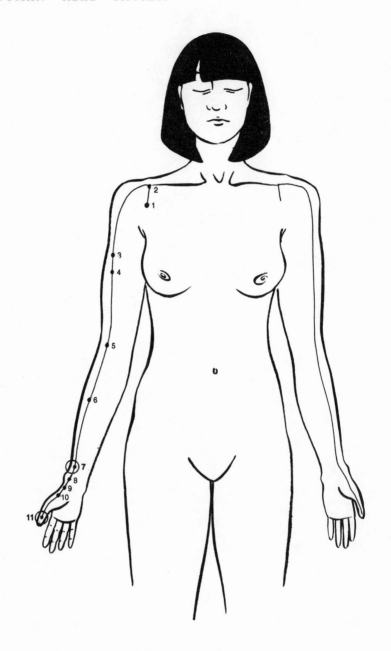

LUNG ENERGY FLOW

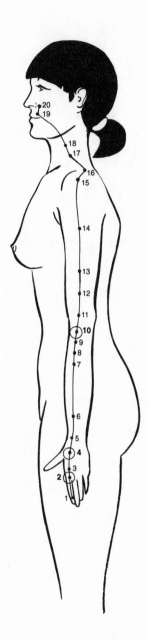

LARGE INTESTINE ENERGY FLOW

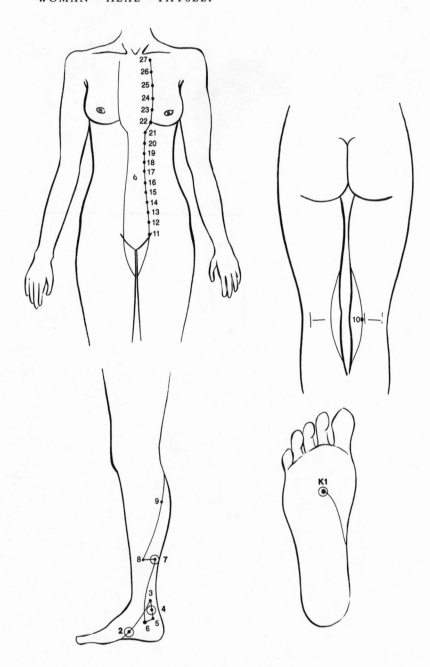

KIDNEY ENERGY FLOW

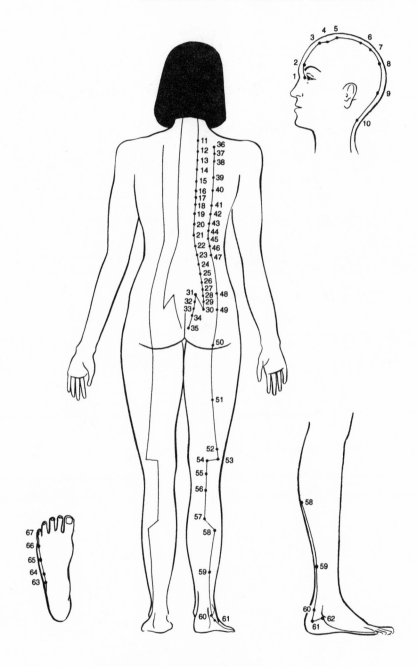

BLADDER ENERGY FLOW

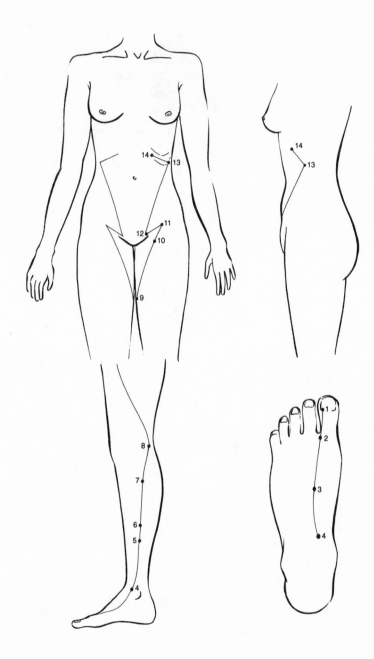

LIVER ENERGY FLOW

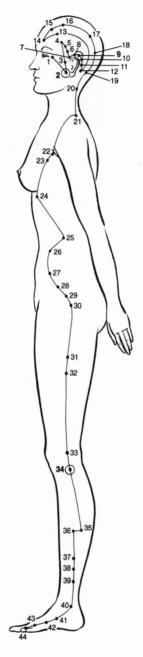

GALLBLADDER ENERGY FLOW

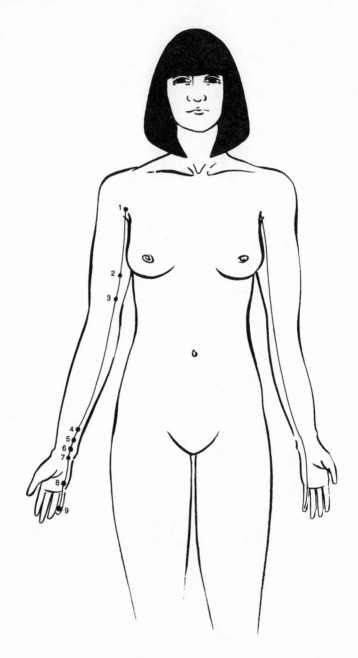

HEART ENERGY FLOW

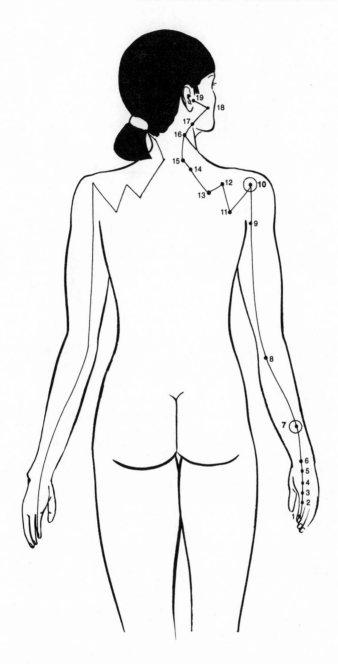

SMALL INTESTINE ENERGY FLOW

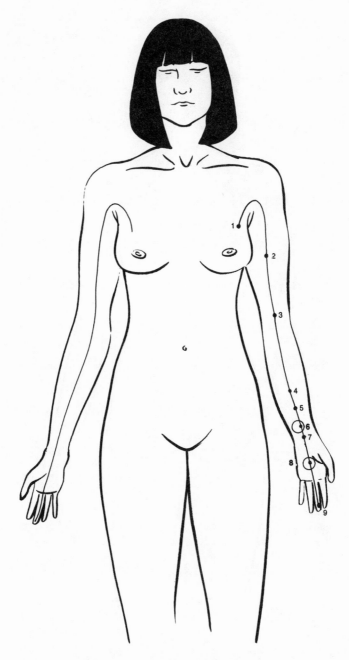

PERICARDIUM ENERGY FLOW

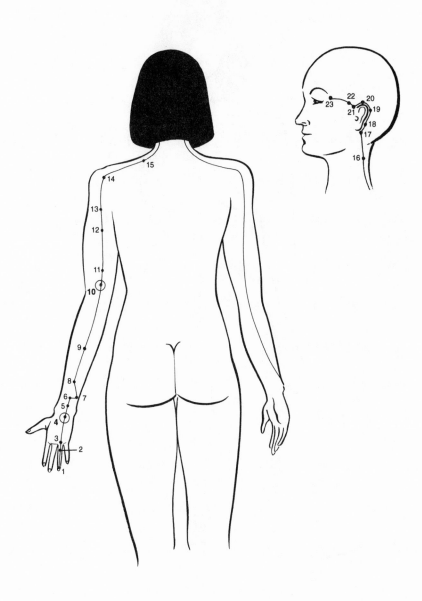

TRIPLE WARMER ENERGY FLOW

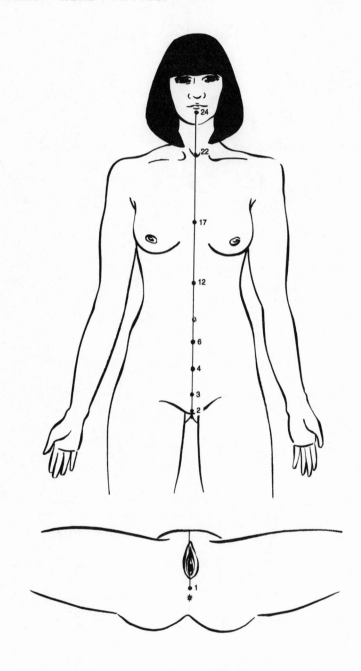

CONCEPTION VESSEL

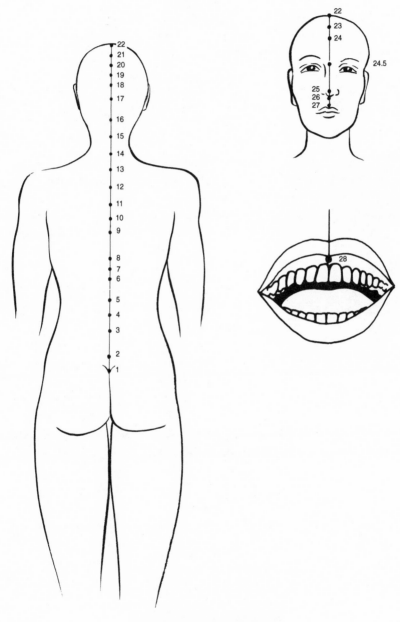

GOVERNING VESSEL

8

 *five element thinking and cycles of energy*

ALTHOUGH WE SPEAK GENERALLY OF "ENERGY," THERE ARE different levels of this energy. We were born with "spirit energy," energy that determines our health (prenatal energy). Then there is energy that we acquire after birth (postnatal energy) through our environment and our family life, and from what we eat, breathe, and drink. So we have the concept of spirit energy and physical energy: *Jing* energy from eating, which is stored in the kidneys; and *Shen* energy from breathing, which is stored in the heart, and associated with spirit, the mind, and emotions.

In the Chinese version of the Creation story, the Creator began by manifesting the Earth. Heaven and Earth became unified, Yin and Yang evolved, and the unity gave birth to the Five Seasons[1], and the Five Elements.

The Five Elements involved in the Oriental system of thought and medical theory are Earth, Metal, Water, Wood, and Fire. The ancient Chinese characterized every aspect of the world into one of these elements and, consequently, each of the major body organs—spleen, stomach, lungs, large intestine, kidneys, bladder, liver, gallbladder, heart, and small intestine—is associated with an element. The Five Elements also became

1. The Five Seasons are Indian Summer, Autumn, Winter, Spring, and Summer.

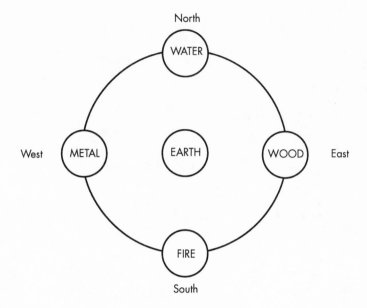

Five Element Chart

known as the Five Movements or the Five Crossroads, and sometimes the Five Phases.

So in addition to all things being either Yin or Yang, they could also be associated with an element. For example, Bladder is Yang, but it is also Water element.

Five Element thinking helps us to see how energy moves and crisscrosses throughout the body. The ancients used the Five Elements to understand how the energies from Heaven and Earth affected human well-being. Health problems were treated using Five Element Theory as a guideline.

The relationships of the Five Elements can be viewed in the diagram above. Within the sequence of energy flow among the Five Elements, Earth was placed in the center and the other elements were positioned on the four principle compass points of north, south, east, and west. Such an arrangement shows us the possible cycles of energy. The relationship of the Five Elements has to do with the giving, taking, and controlling of energy. These cycles of energetic flow are known as the

Birthing Cycle, the Destructive Cycle, and the Controlling Cycle. When these patterns of energy flow are disturbed, chaos results in the physical body. Let's look more closely at these cycles of energy.

The following charts show these three different cycles of energy flow among the Five Elements. Often presented in modern texts as a single conglomeration of circles and arrows, once separated into a series of charts, as I've done here, the energy exchanges can be viewed in stages.

The Birthing Cycle

ON THE MAIN CIRCLE there are arrows pointing in a clockwise direction to indicate the flow of energy in a balanced, healthy person. The Birthing Cycle is a giving cycle.

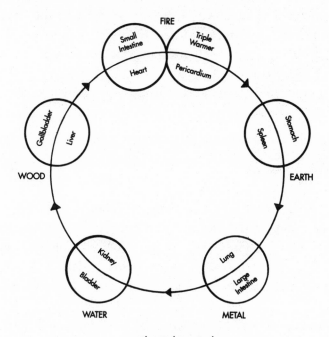

The Birthing Cycle

Earth gives energy to Metal, which gives energy to Water, which gives energy to Wood, which gives energy to Fire, which gives energy back to Earth. In other words, if you want to grow a tree, water it; if you need to burn a fire, put wood on it; for good soil, add ashes; from rich earth, comes metal; to carry water, use a metal container. This is the way the ancients symbolically spoke about the energetic and harmonious flow of the body's energy.

In a healthy, balanced individual, each organ gives energy to the one on its immediate left on the chart. According to Oriental thinking, Water gives life to—or "births," or is the "parent" of—Wood. Wood is the "child" of Water. Each element, in turn, is child, parent, grandchild, and grandparent to another element. This is known as the "parent rule."

Or, reading from an organ point of view, Spleen/Stomach (Earth) give energy to Lung/Large Intestine (Metal), which in turn give energy to Kidney/Bladder (Water), which give energy to Liver/Gallbladder (Wood) and so on through the system if it is healthy and balanced. When an organ is unbalanced in energy, it either has too much energy and is "excessive," or it has too little energy and is "deficient."

It is when imbalance occurs that variations can arise; this often leads to illness.

The Destructive Cycle

WHEN THE CLOCKWISE flow of energy is reversed, the energetic imbalance results in the Destructive Cycle.

Earth destroys Fire, which destroys Wood, which destroys Water, which destroys Metal, which destroys Earth. Or, earth will put out a fire, fire burns wood, wood soaks up water, water rusts metal.

Again, on the level of organs, if there is too much energy

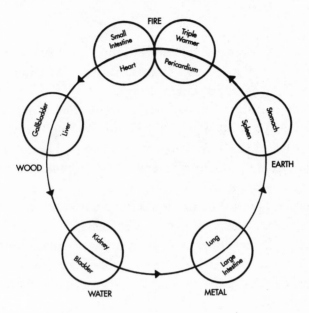

The Destructive Cycle

in Gallbladder/Liver, it can also create an excess in Bladder/Kidney, because Gallbladder/Liver has too much energy and is unable to receive from Bladder/Kidney as it should. This situation can be likened to an unruly child who cannot hear the parent's logic.

Or if Gallbladder/Liver is too low in energy, it can cause Bladder/Kidney to be low as well because of its constant pull for more energy. Like the child for whom any amount of attention is never enough.

There is a third situation that can arise. If Gallbladder/Liver is very weak in energy, it can cause an excess in Bladder/Kidney because Gallbladder/Liver is too weak to receive nourishment, so an excess builds up in the "parent" organ. Like the child who has been hurt or abandoned and for whom comfort has come too late.

The Controlling Cycle

The last set of energetic variations to the Parent rule, illustrated with the Inner Flow Arrows chart, deals with the Grandparent, or Controlling aspect of organ energy.

Earth controls Water, Water controls Fire, Fire controls Metal, Metal controls Wood, and Wood controls Earth. Or we can use earth to block or dam a river, water will dampen a fire, fire is used to melt and purify metal, and metal will prune a tree. It is subtle energy management. The way a grandparent would gently take a grandchild and teach the child values to live by.

If Spleen/Stomach is excessive in energy it will take energy from Bladder/Kidney; an overly doting grandparent who drains the grandchild of affection. Or a deficient Bladder/Kidney will cause a further excess of energy in Spleen/Stomach.

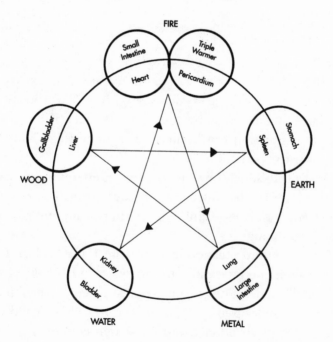

The Controlling Cycle

The unreachable grandchild who infuriates the grandparent by refusing advice.

Or when Bladder/Kidney energy is excessive, it can pull energy from Spleen/Stomach. Similar to a tug-of-war situation where a grandchild push-pulls the grandparent for permission to play at an inappropriate time, the hyperactive grandchild runs circles around the grandparents. A simple problem can have a domino effect on the whole body and disease eventually results, sometimes taking decades to physically manifest.

Within this element system, you will have noticed that the organs are paired, one a female (Yin) organ and the other a male (Yang) organ. In pairs, these organs also affect one another. So if Spleen is excessive with energy, Stomach will have less energy as a balance factor, and vice versa, the way a see-saw works.

The more you study the diagrams, the easier it will be for you to visualize and relate to the body as an energetic flowchart. Or think of it as a family unit of child, parent, and grandparent. The parent organ works to give energy to and sustain life in the child organ, which is controlled by the grandparent organ. Each organ in turn plays a different family role.

Traditional Associations of the Five Elements

Each of the Five Elements has corresponding associations in many different subject areas such as: color, season, compass direction, climate, astrological sign, planet, number, emotional and mental function, body part and opening, smell and taste relating to organ imbalance, animal, moon phase, foods and herbs. The following are the traditional associations. They are listed like this so that they will slip into your unconscious for you to assimilate and draw upon. Note that where Western astrological sun signs are listed, the Chinese moon sign equivalent has been bracketed. The Chinese horoscope animal symbols differ from the traditional Five Element animal associations mentioned from time to time throughout this book.

EARTH: yellow, Indian Summer, humid moisture, center of earth, Earth, number five, spleen-Cancer [Sheep], stomach-Gemini [Horse], mouth, taste, saliva, muscle tone and flesh, lips, mouth, fragrant, sweet, ideas and opinions, intellectual, pensive, sympathy, mindless humming, singing, belching, nourishment, digestion, distribution of nourishment, dates and figs, mallow, millet, lotus, carrots, tofu, pumpkins, winter squash, yam, pear, cherry, cantaloupe, licorice, cinnamon, marjoram, nutmeg, honey, sugar, oxen, Yellow Dragon [ancient], transition, late afternoon, obscured moon, maturity.

METAL: white, Autumn, dry, west, Venus, number nine, lung-Aries [Dragon], large intestine-Taurus [Snake], nose, smell, mucous, skin, rank or rotten, pungent or spicy, lower animal inferior, vitality, grief, weeping or wailing, coughing, breathing, storage and elimination of waste, peach, onion, rice, fennel, radish, ginger, garlic, sesame, skin and bark of many vegetables, blackberry, strawberry, raspberry, mint, cumin, oregano, mustard, curry, cayenne, horse, White Tiger [ancient], quietly sleeping, dusk, decreasing half-moon, harvest gathering, aging.

WATER: blue (or black), Winter, cold, north, Mercury, number six, bladder-Libra [Dog], kidney-Scorpio [Boar], ears, hearing, urine and spittle, bones and marrow, head hair, genitals and anus, putrid, salty, ambition and willpower, will, fear, awe, groan, tremble, energy storage, sexual energy and excretion, fluid, chestnuts, coarse greens, beans, seaweeds, aduki beans, black beans, parsley, apples, walnuts, bindweed, miso, tamari, soy, sea salt, pig, Black Tortoise [ancient], deep slumber, midnight, new moon, hibernation and storage, death.

WOOD: green, Spring, wind, east, Jupiter, number eight, liver-Pisces [Rabbit], gallbladder-Aquarius [Tiger], eyes, sight, tears, tendons and ligaments, muscles and sinews, nails, rancid, sour, soul, spirituality, anger, shout, control, purify, detox, decision-making, plums, leeks, wheat, hemp, new green leafy vegetables, sprouts; white beans, navy beans, and lima beans, green peas, lettuce, pomegranate, sour apples, citrus, valerian, rosemary, basil, vinegar, liquor, oil and fat, fowl, Green Dragon [ancient], awakening, dawn, increasing half-moon, birth.

FIRE: red, Summer, hot, south, Mars, number seven, heart-Leo [Monkey], small intestine-Virgo [Rooster], pericardium-Sagittarius, Triple Warmer-Capricorn, tongue, speech and touch, perspiration, blood vessels, complexion, ears, scorched, bitter, spirit, inspiration, joy, laugh, capability for sadness and grief, insight, sifting pure from impure, intimate relationships, temperature balance, apricots and almonds, scallions, corn, older roots, older greens, burdock, dandelion root, wild greens, rhubarb, mugwort, coriander, thyme, coffee, sheep, Scarlet Bird [ancient], midday, wakefulness, full moon, growth, adulthood.

By using these associations as clues to a puzzle, the ancients could determine which organ or energy flow was out of balance. For example, delving into the Earth associations for a bit of a deeper look, we have "mindless humming" listed. Mindless humming, no tune, no song, just a strange sort of humming, would indicate an imbalance of Spleen, one of the Earth organs. It's a clue. To hum in this manner could be an indication someone is about to dive into a regret-induced cycle of depression, addictions, and rage. It's a red flag. The person can become locked into this humming cycle as a way to control and cover a mounting panic over out of control spiraling thoughts. An "obscured moon" is the phase of the moon which governs the Earth organs. "Muscle tone and flesh" are governed by the Earth organs and problems with the Spleen, in particular, will show up in the muscles or flesh—muscle cramps, sagging muscles, flesh which has lost its elasticity. "Dates and figs" would be good if you wished to boost energy in your Earth organs.

Color in your charts in the Five Element colors. Let them become imprinted in your memory.

The ancients believed in daily meditation, sitting quietly with hands on knees, breathing in through the nose, out through the mouth, visualizing the air from Heaven coming into the body at the back of the neck and traveling down to the feet, energizing the navel area along the way. They advised not to complain about circumstances or to compare or condemn or criticize, but always to think pleasant thoughts and speak good things. They believed that in balancing the five Yin organs, the Heart would become calm, and proper health would occur. All this is explained by Sun Simiao in the *Qiaoji Yao Fang*.

9

twenty-four hours of energy flow

THE ENTIRE FLOW OF ORGAN-ASSOCIATED ENERGY MOVES throughout the body, from one organ to the next, during a twenty-four-hour period.

Each of the twelve primary energy flows has its own peak two-hour time slot, as shown in the chart on page 68. An organ will be at its lowest level of energy (and most vulnerable to disease, illness, or imbalance), exactly twelve hours after it has been at its peak level. I have found that knowing and being mindful of these peak hours has helped me immensely in understanding the way I am feeling physically and emotionally.

Here are some statistical examples of the times organ disease or vulnerability has been most likely to occur in the American population:

More heart attacks happen around noon and many heart failures happen before midnight.

People who have a weak bladder will often have to get up during the night to urinate, usually between 3 and 5 A.M.

The large intestine's peak hours are from 5 to 7 A.M., and it is the early morning when most people have their first bowel movement of the day.

Stomach indigestion most often occurs between 7 and 9

FLOW	PEAK HOUR	LOW HOUR	TYPE
Stomach	7–9 A.M.	7–9 P.M.	Yang
Spleen	9–11 A.M.	9–11 P.M.	Yin
Heart	11–1 P.M.	11–1 A.M.	Yin
Small Intestine	1–3 P.M.	1–3 A.M.	Yang
Bladder	3–5 P.M.	3–5 A.M.	Yang
Kidney	5–7 P.M.	5–7 A.M.	Yin
Pericardium	7–9 P.M.	7–9 A.M.	Yin
Triple Warmer	9–11 P.M.	9–11 A.M.	Yang
Gallbladder	11–1 A.M.	11–1 P.M.	Yang
Liver	1–3 A.M.	1–3 P.M.	Yin
Lung	3–5 A.M.	3–5 P.M.	Yin
Large Intestine	5–7 A.M.	5–7 P.M.	Yang

P.M. after an evening meal and when the stomach is at its lowest energy level. Some schools of thought recommend eating a substantial lunch and a *really* light supper, even going so far as to advise against eating any solid food after 6 P.M. The best time to eat a good hearty breakfast is between 7 and 9 A.M., when the stomach is at its peak energy period.

Have you ever woken from a deep sleep, between 3 and 5 A.M., with tears streaming down your cheeks, your pillow wet, aware that you were crying while you slept, and yet you cannot recall your dream or know why you were weeping? Don't worry, you are just getting rid of some old deeply remembered sorrow during Lung's peak hour, dumping and releasing something you no longer need to hold onto. The lungs physically release grief and sorrow from the body.

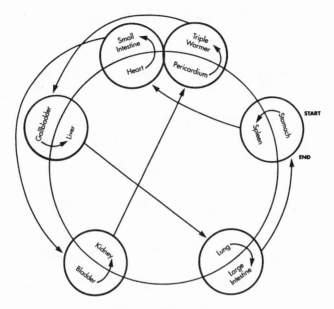

Direction of Flow Chart

Another way I like to look at the peak and low times of the energy flow is to say that it is an energy exchange from partner organ to partner organ and between different generations of the same sex.

In the diagram above, the energy can be explained this way, beginning with the Earth organs of the stomach and spleen.

• Yang Stomach passes the energy to its Yin partner, Spleen.

• Spleen is the Yin daughter of her Yin mother, Heart, and Spleen passes the energy on to Heart.

• Heart passes the energy to her Yang partner, Small Intestine.

• Small Intestine is the Yang grandson of his Yang grandfather, Bladder, and Small Intestine passes the energy to Bladder.

• Bladder passes the energy to his Yin partner, Kidney.

• Kidney is the Yin grandmother of her Yin granddaughter, Pericardium, and Kidney passes the energy on to Pericardium.

• Pericardium passes the energy on to her Yang partner, Triple Warmer.

• Triple Warmer is the Yang son of his Yang father, Gallbladder, and Triple Warmer passes the energy on to Gallbladder.

• Gallbladder passes the energy on to his Yin partner, Liver.

• Liver is the Yin granddaughter of her Yin grandmother, Lung, and Liver passes the energy on to Lung (Yin).

• Lung passes the energy to her Yang partner, Large Intestine.

• Large Intestine is the Yang son of his Yang father, Stomach, and Large Intestine passes the energy flow on to Stomach.

And so we are back at the beginning.

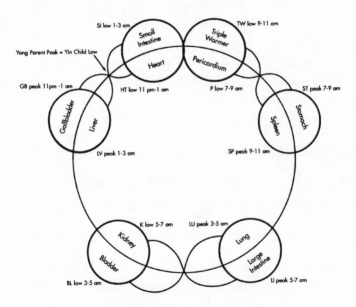

Peak and Low Time Interchange

Another step to understanding the cycle of energy flow is to be aware that when an organ has peak energy it is because it is taking energy from another organ flow.

In these three separate inter-exchange groupings of Spleen/Stomach and Pericardium/Triple Warmer; Lung/Large Intestine and Kidney/Bladder; and Liver/Gallbladder and Heart/Small Intestine, the common factor is that the exchange of energy is from a Yang parent organ to a Yin child organ, and vice versa. For example, when Yang Lung is at peak energy from 3 to 5 A.M. it is taking energy from its Yin child, Bladder, which is at a low energy level between 3 to 5 A.M.

Put these two levels of energy exchange together and this is how the flow of energy works:

• Stomach energy peaks because it pulls energy from Pericardium, which is low in energy.

• Stomach passes peak energy on to Spleen, which peaks because it pulls energy from Triple Warmer, which is low in energy.

• Spleen passes peak energy on to Heart, which peaks because it pulls energy from Gallbladder, which is low in energy.

• Heart passes its peak energy on to Small Intestine, which peaks because it pulls energy from Liver, which is low in energy.

• Small Intestine passes peak energy on to Bladder, which peaks because it pulls energy from Lung, which is low in energy.

• Bladder passes peak energy on to Kidney, which peaks because it pulls energy from Large Intestine, which is low in energy.

• Kidney passes peak energy on to Pericardium, which peaks because it pulls energy from Stomach, which is low in energy.

• Pericardium passes peak energy on to Triple Warmer, which peaks because it pulls energy from Spleen, which is low in energy.

• Triple Warmer passes peak energy on to Gallbladder, which peaks because it pulls energy from Heart, which is low in energy.

• Gallbladder passes peak energy on to Liver, which peaks because it pulls energy from Small Intestine, which is low in energy.

• Liver passes peak energy on to Lung, which peaks because it pulls energy from Bladder, which is low in energy.

• Lung passes peak energy on to Large Intestine, which peaks because it pulls energy from Kidney, which is low in energy.

• Large Intestine passes peak energy on to Stomach, which peaks because it pulls energy from Pericardium.

And once again we are at the beginning of the flow cycle.

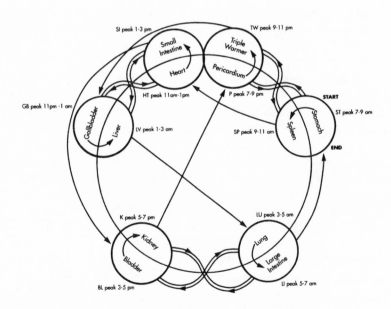

Peaks and Lows of the Twenty-four Hour Flow.

Looking at the timing and interactions between high and low energy of the organs may start you wondering about your day and how patterns can emerge.

For instance, when Pericardium is peaking from 7 to 9 P.M. it is taking energy from Stomach, which is usually busy digesting your dinner at that time. Often people snooze after their evening meal. Why? When we digest our food, the heart works incredibly hard to pump extra blood to the many layers of muscle inside the stomach, which is mulching up the just consumed three-course meal. The pericardium protects the heart, so a snooze actually aids digestion by helping the pericardium conserve energy—by keeping still—while the pericardium is helping the heart as it pumps blood to the stomach for digestion.

The Heart peaks during the usual lunch hours from 11 A.M. to 1 P.M.; this peak period helps again with energy to the stomach for digestion. Small Intestine peaks from 1 to 3 P.M., again aiding with digestion at its most efficient time.

When Large Intestine peaks from 5 to 7 A.M., it is pulling water as well as energy from Kidney. This water goes to the feces in the large intestine and is expelled as the first bowel movement of the day, usually between those hours.

If you are a jogger, fast walker, or like to work out in some way, the best time of day to exercise is from 5-7 P.M. when Kidney—which is the storehouse for all energy—is peaking. You will not only rid the body of stale energy and carbon dioxide through deep breathing (Kidney's natural parent organ is Lung), you will also maximize your exercise efforts by drawing on Kidney at its most efficient time.

The internal time clock of flowing energy can become quite upset when we travel. We call it jet lag. Your Stomach energy is still set to peak between 7 and 9 A.M. But what if you live in Los Angeles and have just flown to London on business? There is an eight-hour time difference. At 3 P.M. in London, your stomach is screaming "Feed me a hearty breakfast!" and what it gets, if it's lucky, is afternoon tea and dainty cucumber sandwiches.

At 7 A.M. the next day, you are attempting to eat your enormous English breakfast while Triple Warmer is still set and peaking at 11 P.M. on your internal clock—it's getting ready to regulate all your energy flows and tuck you into bed back in California. So inside it is still "last night," only now you're in London looking at a plate loaded with eggs and sausages . . . and your eyes are beginning to get very heavy. Which is what you wish they had done at 11 P.M. last night when you had indigestion because Small Intestine was peaking, digestive juices were flowing, ready to digest the lunch that you didn't eat because you were not back in California!

I would have handled the jet lag situation by eating breakfast at 3 P.M. London time—no matter who stared at me—it's what my Stomach wanted. I would have had a light dinner at 7 P.M., because on California time Heart is peaking and can help with blood supply during digestion, and will be tired enough from digestive chores to let me go to bed by 9 P.M. London time. By then, Small Intestine will be peaking on California time, able to help digest both afternoon breakfast and the light supper, while I sleep. All it takes is a little figuring out. With a nice long sleep, my body energy clock would be on London time by the next day.

Chart your own energy highs and lows and notice if you see a pattern emerging from organ to organ. Or track bodily problems throughout the day. Look at the exchange between parent and child energy—Yin and Yang—and see if you pick up any clues about physical organ problems you may have.

10

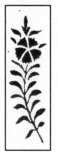 *emotions and the body*

FROM THE LIST OF YIN-YANG ASSOCIATIONS ON PAGES 36 AND 37, you will have noticed that the body organs were also divided into masculine (Yang) and feminine (Yin). Each feminine organ in our body is associated with an emotion, and that particular organ is responsible for dealing with that emotion, processing or "digesting" the emotion, as it were, and releasing it from the physical body. Thoughts and the power of the mind can have a wonderfully strong and positive effect on our physical well-being, or a potentially disastrous negative one. Physical disease really can begin with an imbalance of the emotions.

For example, the Liver is associated with the emotion of anger. When we have unreleased anger, it will go to the Liver. A person may develop an alcohol problem because of a subconscious desire to numb that anger. The effect of the alcohol can then release the anger as the drinker relaxes control of the emotions (Gallbladder is Liver's partner and "Control" is its primary concern), making some people violent while under the influence.

Heart attacks have often been known to take place after dinner, following a heated family argument. The Liver/Gallbladder pair associated with anger and control have taken energy from the Heart/Small Intestine, which require the energy for digestion. The Heart needs energy to pump blood for the digestion process. Walk a mile or eat a large meal—the heart uses roughly the same amount of energy for both activities. Liver pulling energy for the internal anger process, or Gallbladder pulling energy to control the situation and the anger level inside—both take energy from Heart. So on a very basic survival level, no violent arguments over dinner!

The emotion of fear is associated with the Kidneys. Fear can solidify and manifest physically as kidney stones. Many women who have been sexually abused as children (or as adults) often carry kidney and bladder infections all their lives. Fear associated with their abuse goes to this area. Thoughts of shame or guilt will also connect with and collect in the sexual area, often resulting in menstrual problems, cysts, infertility, and tumors. Guilt often results from anger that has been turned inward.

Since the Lungs are associated with grief, if you fail to cry when you feel deep sorrow, that sadness will settle in the lungs and over time will build up. I had a client who had never mourned the death of her husband some years before. As her grief went unexpressed, it began to manifest as breathing problems, and, eventually, a suspicious area appeared in the right lung. She was told it would require a biopsy. She then had a three-hour auricular therapy session with me on the Saturday before the planned biopsy, and we worked all the Lung points in her ear. She wept, sobbed, and grieved her husband's passing and talked about her loneliness without him. On Tuesday, she went in for her planned biopsy, but a prescreen before surgery showed no suspicious area in the lung.

The Gallbladder is associated with control. That can involve any situation where someone is being controlled, controlling, or out of control. Often patients who have had their gallbladders removed experience feeling a loss of control over their lives.

The Spleen processes overconcern, reminiscence, and

worry. Spleen's other half, Pancreas, though not mentioned on the Five Element charts, deals with regret or anxiety. When you dwell on the past—what you did, what you didn't do, what you should have done—you are judging yourself. When you behave in this way, you are generally being so hard on yourself that one of your energy meridians is seriously affected and begins to lose energy very rapidly. It's as though one of your energy circuits is leaving your body. You are engaging in wasted energy. Stop singing "The Would-a, Could-a, Should-a Blues." We can learn from the past.

One of my clients, who lovingly and somewhat playfully refers to himself as "Mr. Regret," used to spend 80 percent of the time bemoaning his past, and nurturing and hanging onto various and numerous regrets. He drove himself into panic and depression wondering why things happened the way they did. "What ifs" rounded out his daily diet. He was a master at making himself miserable: his misery overflowed onto those around him. He had a black belt in regret.

To help Mr. Regret maintain energetic balance, I met with him at least every week, constantly draining off the negative energy that he had accumulated by dwelling on his regrets or focusing on what he wondered might happen in the future "if." Many of his regrets focused on past relationships that failed. He pondered if he should try again, have another go at it, and would reconnect with women from his past, with little regard for his wife, or the women from his past with whom he would toy emotionally.

The regrets collected in his sexual area—because regret is processed by Spleen, which governs the sexual organs—and, as a result, we battled to keep pre-cancerous cells in his prostate gland at bay. Energy medicine will almost never be effective with people like this, because their minds are so undisciplined, so unable to stay focused on living in the present, that their energetic system is overwhelmed and creates chaos in the physical body. They manifest forms of illness beyond the help

of energy work, and the illnesses eventually require traditional allopathic treatment with drugs or surgery. These individuals tend to give energy workers, who attempt to help them, a
bad name. A healing therapist can only help you help heal
yourself.

The Heart and the Pericardium, the sack in which the
heart sits, contend with shock, hurt, and excessive joy. As an
example, there was a woman (let's call her Jane) who walked in
on her husband and a friend having sex.

On this occasion, as Jane drove home in her car, she began
to feel nauseous; her stomach felt like it was attempting to
digest a meal of cement. The closer she got to her house, the
more nauseated she became. When she got home her hand was
shaking as she tried to get the key in the door. Her heart was
pounding so hard, pushing so much blood to her brain, that she
could sense its redness behind her eyes. She knew intuitively
what she'd find: her husband and her friend were naked in the
afternoon sunlight. The guest was mortified at being caught, the
husband only resented her intrusion.

This was the first time in her life that Jane made no
attempt to hold her tongue; she didn't care how foul her lan-
guage was, or who heard her. She didn't try to "make nice."
Obscenities bounced off the walls. She drove to her therapist
screaming abuse and crying, brokenhearted. For over an hour
she sobbed in his office.

Finally, he looked at her very intently and said "I want you
to stay in your anger as you drive home, just stay angry at your
husband and your friend for what they have done." This was
incredibly confusing for Jane; someone was actually giving her
permission to be furious! Upon her return home, she was
indeed still angry and screamed at both of them until she could
yell no longer.

Five months elapsed before the pain of that incident sub-
sided; she even came apart in public a few weeks after the event,
pent up tears of the pain betraying her. She said she felt more

humiliated and shamed by that loss of self-control than by the original adultery.

This trauma, and the months of emotional stress that followed, severely weakened her heart. As she turned the key, her legs were shaking from fear coursing through the Kidney flow; her arms were shaking from energy leaving her body through her Heart flow; her heart was actually emotionally "breaking." Her body was on fire from the anger in her Liver flow as the rage came out. The severe stress took its toll on her physical body because three major flows were involved, Kidney, Liver, and Heart, almost to complete energetic depletion.

One primary cause of stress is the distance between what we say we believe and the way we live our lives.

What if you say you believe in monogamy but you love and live with a man who plays around? How do you think that kind of inner turmoil is going to affect your body over time? The wrinkles around your eyes and the sad look on your face only begin to tell the story. Power struggles over behavioral patterns are emotional abuse issues and will affect your genital organs and the lower abdominal area.

It is the daily betrayals of our own personal belief systems that kill us. They create energetic havoc on a cellular level. Whose belief systems are they anyway—your parents? An uncle? The Church? Is the way you live in synch with the way your Heart wants to live? Does your heart cry out to live in the woods with nature, and yet you live in the desert or a city high-rise? This is what the 90s are asking us to do—get real—live in step with the desires of our Spirit.

The energy flows that I believe to be most important for women are:

• the Spleen, which governs the reproductive system; it is actually the Spleen pulse that is felt to determine pregnancy status.

• the Kidneys, which are the body's storehouse for all energy.

When Kidney energy becomes depleted, sexual energy diminishes—no desire, no lubrication, the "not tonight, darling" syndrome (for men, impotency can result).

• the Large Intestine, because its function is the elimination of impure thoughts, constipation of the mind. Throughout history women have been forced by men to keep quiet, not speak their mind; their opinions were often disregarded, thoughts could not flow.

• the Gallbladder, governing as it does control issues, because women have also been controlled for generations by society in general.

• the Liver, because as a gender we have a great deal of repressed anger to deal with, whether we like to admit it or not.

For hundreds of years, women have been controlled by men—and it has affected the way we dress, sit, speak, and think. Women have generally been regarded as necessary for a few functions, nameable on one hand. Many women have repressed their anger, their frustration, and feel like they are being controlled, have no control over their lives, or cannot do what they want. On the chart of the Five Elements, Gallbladder/Liver are opposite Spleen/Stomach. After a time of overcontrol and suppressed anger, the result can be reproductive or sexual problems: tumors, cysts, infertility, water retention, lowered immunity, loose bowels, and a tired heavy body; all from an imbalanced Spleen. Arthritis (a holding-onto-anger disease), allergies, eye problems, indigestion, soft nails, depression, weight gain, itching, and bruising are all associated with poor Liver energy level.

A friend came to me and said she could not understand how her health could possibly have become so bad so quickly. When I asked her to tell me what was happening in her life, she said that she had been going through a particularly difficult divorce, completely at the mercy of, and controlled (Gallbladder energy flow) by her husband, and that she was furious and felt helpless to do anything about it. She had developed cysts and fibroid tumors on one ovary and many in her uterus (Spleen energy flow); her appetite was poor, and she had a stomach ulcer (Stomach is energy partner of Spleen flow). Look at the chart for progression of depleted energy on page 62. My first thought was to ask if she suffered from kidney or bladder problems. She immediately said "No," then quickly added, "But I've had sties in my eyes lately." She then looked confused and said, "I wonder why I told you that?" Her intuition wanted to give me information that she, on a conscious level, could not understand. One of the interesting aspects of Oriental medicine is that there are places on the body, related to the organs, yet not near them, where symptoms of organ imbalance will show up. The lower eye area is associated with the kidneys.

Although a doctor of Oriental medicine was treating her through herbal teas and acupuncture, and her cysts and fibroid tumors shrank significantly in size (60 percent) over a six-month period, she did eventually opt for a hysterectomy. Now she is in another controlling relationship where she often cannot find words for what she feels, because her sentences are censored if the man in her life does not like what she is saying or finds no merit in her opinion. Her emotions continue to soar and plummet. She says she feels great, but she is losing weight, looks anorexic, and has so much pain in her eyes that I feel like crying for her. Simply put, she is in denial. None of us can force someone to come out of denial, no matter how much we care for them.

Kidneys deal with fear. Grief collects in the Lungs. As little children, sometimes we want to cry and our parents won't let us; or as adults we stop ourselves, because we're grown up and someone might see us. When we want to cry and don't, the suppressed emotion goes to the Lungs. As children, little girls are told it's all right to cry but not to get angry; getting angry is not "ladylike." Little boys are told that it's all right to get mad, but not to cry; crying is not "manly."

In adult life, as a result of conditioned repressed emotional responses, a woman may want to yell when angry, but she bursts into tears instead; the anger stays inside her, and inappropriate tears result. Perhaps she may develop an alcohol problem to numb the repressed anger. A man may want to cry but since childhood he has been programmed against this, so he yells or hits, and the result is inappropriate anger and his grief remains unexpressed. Perhaps he will develop a smoking problem to numb that accumulated grief. In each case, there is incorrect energy flow between Lung and Liver.

What we do to our bodies to suppress our deep-rooted emotions appears endless: smoking; drug-taking; eating disorders—overeating, anorexia nervosa, or bulimia—sexual addiction; physical, sexual, verbal, and emotional abuse of others; becoming alcoholics or social drinkers, kleptomaniacs, compulsive liars, shoppers, or gamblers.

As a society and as a world, we are in a perilous state, the origins of which we can trace back to our feelings, or their suppression, to emotional holes that we try to fill with other people or things, and to greed, power manipulation, selfishness, and totally self-centered behavior on a global basis.

Emotional Give and Take

Expressed in an Oriental manner, here is a synopsis of how the emotions effect our well-being as they progress through the Five Elements.

Spleen that is full of regret, overconcern, and reminiscence, will TAKE energy from Kidney, so that trust, respect, the ability to relax, the desire for self-healing and willpower are impossible. Therefore, Spleen is UNABLE TO GIVE energy to Lung,

so that greed, jealousy, pride, selfishness, envy, self-pity, depriva-
tion, and despondency may result.

Lung that is full of sadness and grief will TAKE energy
from Liver, so that self-assertion and motivation are impossible.
Therefore, Lung is UNABLE TO GIVE energy to Kidney, so
that inferiority, panic, paranoia, mistrust, or feelings of superior-
ity may result.

Kidney that is full of fear and terror will TAKE energy
from Heart, so that joy, self-confidence, compassion, and love
cannot be felt. Therefore, Kidney is UNABLE TO GIVE energy to Liver so that self-blame, guilt, boredom, impotency, frigid-
ity, resentment, bitterness, depression, and non-motivation may
result.

Liver that is full of anger will TAKE energy from Spleen,
so that sympathy and empathy cannot be felt. Therefore, Liver is
UNABLE TO GIVE energy to Heart, so that despair, self-
doubt, hopelessness, nervousness, hysteria, or depression may
result.

Heart that is full of hurt, shock, and shut down, will TAKE
energy from Lung, so that nonattachment, grieving, letting go,
and openness cannot happen. Therefore, Heart is UNABLE TO
GIVE energy to Spleen, so that forgetfulness, mental fatigue,
lack of concentration, worry, obsessiveness, and indifference
may result.

Does any of the above information help you recognize emotional imbalance in yourself? Take a highlighter and outline
words that describe feelings that you have experienced, then
compare the emotions to physical illnesses that you had at one
time or another. What organs were affected? Can you find a pattern to your illnesses? A spiraling down from one form of
imbalance into another?

As children, the majority of us were never taught to have
a relationship with our bodies, let alone our organs. The way of

thinking presented here may take some getting used to. But I assure you, once you become familiar with the interconnection of the organs and the emotional states these organs govern, you will achieve a new understanding of a body you may never have known.

I I

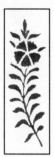

using the five elements to diagnose dis-ease

WE HAVE LOOKED AT THE EFFECTS OF EMOTIONAL IMBALANCE on the physical body. In this chapter we will look at the physical and mental functions associated with each organ. Emotions originate in the right hemisphere of the brain, which controls the left, Yin side of the body. Mental thought and action stem from the left side of the brain, which controls the right, Yang side of the body. If emotional and energetic imbalance occurs, mental function will also be impaired.

Earth Organs

SPLEEN/PANCREAS/STOMACH: Secretions from the pancreas are released into the small intestine and serve to digest proteins, fats, and starches. The Islets of Langerhans—differentiated cell groups within the pancreas—create the hormones insulin and glucogon. The pancreas is vital to our physical nourishment.

An imbalanced Pancreas can manifest physically as weak muscles, pale and dry lips and mouth, diminished taste, swollen knees and thighs, belching, diabetes, abdominal distention, and a heavy, weak, and "achy" feeling to the body. Pancreas is also associated with saliva.

The spleen removes dead red cells from the blood and creates antibodies, which inhibit poisonous bacteria from having an effect on us. The spleen is responsible for the overall health of our immune system. It also acts as the distributor for the energy obtained from food digested by the stomach. It aids in the production of saliva and manifests health or ill health in the lips.

An imbalanced Spleen energy flow can result in sticky feces, sugar cravings, diarrhea, laziness, need to sleep or lie down too much, joint pain, infrequent urination, constipation, appetite problems, hypoglycemia, pale skin, pain or discomfort in the big toe, nausea after eating, swollen abdomen, flatulence, memory loss, and a heavy achy feeling in the legs.

The Spleen is responsible for energetically supporting the mental function of all other energy flows.

The stomach deals with digestion. Without a properly functioning stomach and proper extraction of nutrients, the entire body system will soon have problems. The stomach also affects the salivary glands. When we vomit, the Stomach energy is reversed and flows backwards (or upwards).

An imbalanced Stomach flow will show up in lip and mouth sores, swollen gums, nose bleeds, runny or stuffy nose, dark patches on the face, restlessness, frequent yawning, thoughts of food, pain when swallowing due to a swollen esophagus, the ability to be easily startled, bad breath, leg cramps, numbing pain in the second toe, abdominal distention, gluttonous hunger and thirst or loss of appetite, dark yellow urine, workaholic and antisocial behavior.

The mental function of the Stomach has to do with the "digestion" of thoughts.

Metal Organs

LUNGS/LARGE INTESTINE: The lungs regulate the way we breathe. They absorb the energy (from heaven) in the air and

extract oxygen from it to oxygenate our blood. Lung is associated with the skin and with body hair, which regulates the body
temperature in times of severe cold or heat. Lung is also associated with mucus, the nose, and smell.

An imbalanced Lung energy flow may result in loss of
smell, insomnia, poor resistance to coughs and colds, noisy bowels with diarrhea, afternoon fever, voice loss, excessive phlegm,
wet dreams, claustrophobia, little urine passed with a great urge
present, cold limbs or hot palms, upper back and arm aches,
weak thumbs, and an overactive sex drive.

The mental function of Lung is to absorb good thoughts.

The large intestine, or colon, eliminates excess matter from
the digestive process. Constipation will eventually lead to a
buildup of toxins in the whole system if not alleviated.

Imbalanced Large Intestine energy may manifest in arm
and shoulder pain, nosebleeds, toothaches and gum disease, constipation, diarrhea, voice loss, inability to feel joy, shivering, sore
throat, orange urine, excessive thirst with a dry mouth, dizziness, distended abdomen, sore or itching or other index finger
problems, sad and gloomy outlook on life, shivering and a feeling of still being cold even after warming up.

The mental function of Large Intestine has to do with the
elimination of impure thoughts.

Water Organs

KIDNEY/BLADDER: The Kidneys are the storehouse of all
extra energy and distribute it back to other organs as they
require it. From this stored energy (Jing) comes the ability of
the testicles and ovaries to produce sperm and eggs. Lack of
Kidney energy is equal to lack of sexual energy. The Kidneys are
also associated with the ears and hearing; the bones and bone
marrow, which produces red blood cells; the brain and the
adrenal and parathyroid glands. The kidneys regulate salt balance

in the water of the bloodstream and filter out substances not required after the digestion of food.

An imbalance in Kidney flow can result in an astonishing array of ailments: hunger with anorexia, irregular menstruation, hoarse voice, tinnitus (ringing in the ears), diarrhea, premature senility, aching bones, restless sleep, balding, drowsiness, blurring of vision, constant fear, fear of the dark, impotency, lumbago, excessive sexual desire, lack of willpower, cold feet and legs, pain in the sole of the foot, urinary incontinence, dry tongue and hot mouth, sore swollen throat yet no cold or cough, over-sensitivity to cold, and pain or heat in the soles of the feet.

The mental function of Kidney is an open mind and clarity of thought.

The Bladder energy flow begins in the inner corner of the eye, moves through the forehead, across the top of the head, down the back and into the legs and feet. It plays a large part in balance between body and mind. Mind strain will often accumulate in the buttocks, lower back, between the shoulder blades and neck area, causing severe pain. Physically, the bladder is in charge of creating a proper fluid level in the body and encourages the kidneys to function; it receives and excretes urine produced by the kidneys.

Imbalances of this flow can cause lumbar pain, small toe pain, clear nasal discharge, bladder irritation or burning, spasms in the calf muscle, dry eyes, protruding eyeballs, eye pain, cloudy urine, sciatica, neuralgia, narcolepsy, lack of balance, pain behind the knees, headaches at the eyebrow and top of the head, bedwetting, urinary incontinence, lack of movement in the hip, and tight knee muscles.

My father's nose was very badly shattered in an accident when he was in his early twenties. This interfered with the beginning point of his Bladder and Stomach energy flows, and it began to affect him physically. First, toward the end of every meal, clear fluid would pour from his sinuses. Shortly after this problem began, he developed narcolepsy. Then hip problems plagued him for no "known" reason. In his mid-sixties he was stricken with bladder cancer, which eventually spread to his kidneys eleven years later and resulted in his death. No allopathic doctor ever connected any of these physical problems with a root cause of energetic imbalance, and he was treated by some of the best in the world. Unfortunately and sadly, he never ventured into the world of Oriental medicine to seek a cure for his ills.

The mental function of the Bladder is to eliminate impure ideas.

Wood Organs

LIVER/GALLBLADDER: The liver secretes the bile that is stored in its partner organ, the gallbladder. Bile is necessary for the digestion of soluble fats which contain vitamins A, D, E, and K. The liver filters the blood from the stomach, spleen, and intestines, helps to regulate the blood sugar level and stores starch, releasing it as sugar as the body requires it. The liver neutralizes various poisons, including drugs and alcohol. Liver also helps to control the nervous system and plays a part in brain function as related to anger and depression, which can become clinical depression (having a biochemical basis) if allowed to go on for too long.

If Liver flow is out of balance, a person may suffer from allergies, bruise easily, have either very soft or hard nails, testicular pain, premenstrual tension, vertigo, irritability and bad temper, large toe problems, indigestion and gas, water retention, over acidity, bed-wetting, eye problems (including difficulty looking down or up), insomnia, extreme depression, muscular cramps and spasms, yellowing of the whites of the eyes, and itching. Sexual problems can also result, such as swelling of the penis, a lack of erection, an altogether excessive erection, and orgasmic dysfunction in women. The Liver "houses the human soul, which is said to enter the foetus at the moment of birth."[1]

The mental function of the Liver is foresight and planning.

The gallbladder stores bile and secretes it into the duodenum (part of the small intestine) by contracting itself during digestion. If the gallbladder is weak, it will not secrete enough bile, which primarily breaks down fats, so that fatty or fried foods may cause problems.

Imbalances in Gallbladder flow may result in migraine headaches, bitter mouth taste, stiff muscles and joint pain, vertigo, thyroid or arm pit tumors, hearing difficulties, jaw pain, rib and chest pain, quickness to anger, deafness, weak tendons in the legs, eye pain, soft bones, sciatica, frequent sighing, pain in the small toe or outside of foot, weak legs, irritability or timidity.

The mental function of Gallbladder is judgment control and decision making.

Fire Organs

HEART/SMALL INTESTINE and PERICARDIUM/ TRIPLE WARMER: The Heart regulates all other energy flows and must be strong for the body and emotions to be healthy. The heart pumps the blood and regulates the blood vessels. Our Spirit dwells in the heart; our mental clarity and emotional moods are said to come from the heart.

When Heart flow is imbalanced there may be insomnia, hysteria, swollen tongue, high blood pressure, red nose, night sweats, hot flashes, dark urine, fitful sleep, cold sweats, numbing of the tongue, chest pain, palpitations, dizziness, dull nipple pain, confusion, pale tongue, red tongue, pains in the inner arm, speech problems, or dry mouth and throat.

1. Daniel P. Reid, *Chinese Herbal Medicine* (Boston: Shambhala Publications, 1993), p. 34.

The mental function of Heart is to coordinate all other aspects of mental function.

The small intestine assimilates food before it passes into the large intestine; it controls the amount of liquid in the feces and regulates the amount of water that is passed out for elimination or reabsorption into the body.

Imbalance in Small Intestine flow can lead to a hard distended abdomen, bursitis, shoulder pain, reddish urine, temple headaches, tinnitus, inability to gain weight, weak arms, pain in the little finger, diarrhea alternating with constipation, undigested food in the feces, immobile neck, and late menstrual periods. Blood in the urine results when the heart gets overheated, the small intestine's water regulation is inhibited, and kidney function suffers.

The mental function of Small Intestine is to discriminate between impure and pure thoughts.

The pericardium, the permeable sack that encloses the heart, is lubricated to prevent friction as the heart beats. It also protects the heart emotionally, so that a weak Heart would indicate a weak Pericardium as well. Pericardium flow also deals with emotional sexuality and is sometimes called the "Circulation Sex Meridian." It controls the sexual function of Kidney energy and deals with the real "Self" and with relationships of the Heart.

An imbalanced Pericardium flow can result in hot palms, stiff arm and elbow, dull eyes, constraint in the throat, swollen arm pit, high blood pressure, indigestion, light sleep, elbow spasm, heart discomfort, excessive dreaming, encephalitis, pain in the arms, chest distention, stiff head and neck, pain in the middle finger, red face and chest, lack of joy or sexual energy, and incessant laughter or forced laughter.

The mental function of Pericardium is to support one's self-worth.

The Triple Warmer regulates the energy between all other flows and is thought to be energetically linked to the hypothalamus, which is the bridge between the endocrine glands and the nervous system.

Triple Warmer imbalance will often result in problems with social relationships, ring finger pain, appetite, thirst, abnormal sugar levels, wakefulness, low back pain, throat infections, abdominal distention, cold and fevers, memory loss, mental confusion, eye pain, tight jaw, deafness, temple headaches, high and low mood swings, throat obstruction, cold hands and feet, urinary dysfunction, and perspiration for no reason.

The mental function of Triple Warmer is to nurture and sustain family relationships.

The Curious Organs

In addition to the traditional organs previously discussed, there are six additional organs that do not come into play for diagnostic purposes. They are mentioned in the *Nei Ching—The Yellow Emperor's Classic of Internal Medicine*. I present them here only for reference. You might find it of interest if, say, in addition to the symptoms you are already tracking, you notice changes in one or more of these areas as well. You may then want to follow up with more advanced study of Oriental medicine.

The six Curious Organs are the Bones, the Uterus, the Marrow, the Blood Vessels, the Brain and, curiously enough, the Gallbladder. The Gallbladder is a Yang organ involved with digestion and also classified as a Curious Organ because it produces a substance, bile. The Curious Organs are considered to have been created by the Earth and are Yin in form.[2]

Imbalances of the Bones, Marrow, and Brain are generally treated through the Kidney meridian; the Uterus through the Spleen, Liver, and Kidney Flows; the Blood by way of the Heart, Spleen, and Liver.

2. Ted J. Kaptchuck, *The Web that Has No Weaver* (Chicago: Congdon and Weed, 1993), p. 34.

The Miscellaneous Flows

As previously mentioned at the beginning of chapter 7, the only two Miscellaneous Flows we will be considering are the Governing Vessel, which is Yang, and the Conception Vessel which is Yin. Both of these channels have their own specific points on the body and also intersect with different major flows. They have a close connection with and effect on several of the Curious Organs. They are referred to as "Vessels" because they do not flow as the other meridians do, but store energy and regulate the other flows by giving energy as needed.

THE GOVERNING VESSEL is classed as a Yang meridian. It is said to govern the six Yang flows—Stomach, Large Intestine, Bladder, Gallbladder, Small Intestine, and Triple Warmer—which join at Governing Vessel 14 (see page 55). The Governing Vessel is particularly important because it moves into the spine, then enters and nourishes the brain, and is responsible for spinal fluid quality. It also connects with the kidneys, which are the storehouse for all sexual energy, so it has a direct effect upon sexual function.

Any imbalance in this vessel can lead to mental malfunction, dizziness, infertility, back pain, hemorrhoids, constipation, acute pain in the bowels, dark colored urine, numbing of the legs, vaginal discharge, rectal prolapse, diarrhea, epilepsy, premature ejaculation, poor or worsening vision, memory loss, headaches, cardiac pain, voice loss, jaundiced eyes or body, jaw tightness, nasal polyps, insomnia, acute drowsiness, madness, facial sores, tinnitus, bleeding gums, swollen face, runny nose, nosebleeds, impotence, no perspiration, knee pain, drooling, irregular menstruation, and dry tongue.

THE CONCEPTION VESSEL: The Conception Vessel is considered Yin, and three Yin flows—Liver, Spleen, and Kidney—meet in this meridian at various points. It has two routes, one up the back in the spine and one up the front of the body. It joins Stomach Flow 1 and Governing Vessel 28 during its passage up the back, and is said to regulate all Yin flows, pregnancy, and the fetus. The Conception Vessel and the Governing Vessel store extra Kidney energy, which, if they are in balance, regulate the menstrual flow each month.

Imbalances of the Conception Vessel are said to cause infertility, irregular menstruation, lack of menstruation, white vaginal discharge (leukorrhea), genital itching or swelling, uterine prolapse, dizziness, diarrhea, seminal emissions, dark urine, edema, open fontanels in babies, nosebleeds, rectal prolapse, vomiting, abdominal distension, appetite loss, taste loss, jaundice, smell loss, manic rage, memory loss, constipation, anxiety/panic attacks, chest pain, back pain, mouth sores, tight jaws, emotional withdrawal, epilepsy, heart palpitations, and swollen pharynx.

IN ORDER TO BECOME aware of your physical/mental/emotional symptoms and the organ flow involved, you will need to chart what is going on on a daily basis. Keep a journal, or make a quick list before you retire for bed:

"*Tuesday: headache at 10 A.M.—lunch with Susan, bowel spasms again—worked overtime (deadlines to meet!)—pain running down front of left leg—craving sweets—trouble falling asleep.*"

Do the same thing for Wednesday, or every other day, or as often as fits into your lifestyle. Make sure you list everything that has an impact on you, regardless of whether it's physical, emotional, or mental. Eventually, certain patterns will emerge. Check the lists of associations (pages 63-65) for the elements and the organ flows involved. Start by looking at the relationships. Which organ flows are involved? Which elements? Are you noticing any patterns? Are the same organ flows involved even if the symptoms change? Look up specific symptoms in the "Diagnostic Reference" in Part Five, and see which energy flows are involved.

Are you noticing that most of what you are charting falls under the heading of Earth? Water? Perhaps a couple of elements are consistently involved. When you add up the symptoms, how many are Yin? Yang?

Refer back to chapter 8, "Cycles of Energy." Can you detect a particular cycle of energy into which your symptoms fall? Does your energy seem to be backing up, or moving in a destructive cycle?

It will take some time for you to become comfortable thinking about your body in terms of Chinese medicine. As you progress, you'll discover that self-awareness and your own intuition will be the greatest allies in healing yourself.

12

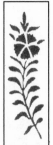 *the nature of pain—or, why does it hurt?*

PAIN IS THE BODY'S WAY OF WARNING US THAT SOMETHING IS wrong. Never ignore pain. It means we have either hurt ourselves, have an illness or a disease, or that an imbalance within an energy flow has actually manifested as physical discomfort.

Allopathic—Western—doctors often refer to these energetic types of pain as "psychosomatic." There is the implication that the pain is in the patient's mind, and that it is actually unreal. In the allopathic world, the pain is untreatable and the belief is it will eventually "go away," usually after the patient stops worrying about the "problem." The patient may even be given some kind of placating medication, such as a painkiller or anti-inflammatory drug.

Traditional Oriental Medicine, on the other hand, takes all types of pain very seriously. Pain, too, can be classified into a Yang or Yin type. This is helpful in locating the problem organ or organ flow involved in the discomfort.

Yang Associated Pain

Pain that is Yang in origin tends to be new, acute, and can come and go. It is made worse by pressure, warmth, movement; the skin may be red, dry, and hot to the touch. The pain may be eased when exposed to cold and may also wander from its point of origin. It is usually throbbing, shallow, precisely defined, strangling, spasming, hard to the touch, and can come on fairly quickly.

Depending on the ailment, the pain may be accompanied by insomnia, possibly with disturbing thoughts. There may be a desire for a light sunny room, out of the darkness, the eyes may be restless and lacking focus with a tendency to wander. The mouth may be dry, and you may crave salt. Noisy expression of the pain, such as moaning, groaning, crying out, and bed covers thrown off, are symptoms and behavior patterns that signify a Yang type of problem.

Yin Associated Pain

Pain that is Yin in origin tends to be old or chronic. It is worsened by exposure to cold; the skin may be clammy, damp with perspiration, pale, and cold to the touch. Yin pain may be alleviated by movement, warmth, and pressure, and is fixed and constant in its location. It is usually widespread, deep, or heavy. There could be bruising or pain in the bones, and the area may be flaccid to the touch.

Depending on the ailment, the pain may be accompanied by a strange deep sleep state where dreaming and thoughts are present yet difficult to recall or grasp. The eyes may be sensitive to light; eyes half shut, lifeless, and staring. Excessive salivation, sugar craving, desire for rigid silence, an inability to discuss the pain or ailment, and depression and listlessness may be present.

ONCE YOU HAVE determined to the best of your ability whether the pain you are experiencing is predominantly Yang or Yin, notice which physical organ is in the area, or what organ flow runs through the pain. Physical organ? Energetic flow?

Let's look at some examples of pain. Why do so many women also suffer from pains in their legs, along with low tummy cramps, during their menstrual period? After all, the uterus is not located in the thigh! This thigh pain is more than likely due to a blockage of energy along the Spleen Flow; energy which should be releasing during menstruation is backed up, often causing very real, debilitating pain.

Migraine headaches are classified in Oriental terms as being associated with overactive Liver energy. This type of energy is called "rising," or traditionally called Hyper Liver Yang Ascending. The Yang aspect of the Yin Liver organ is excessive. If you look at the body chart for Liver flow (on page 48), you will see it is nowhere near the head. However, where is its partner organ, Gallbladder flow (page 49), located? The head. What other part of the body is Liver associated with? The eyes. Migraines are usually throbbing, accompanied by dizziness, blurred vision, and often nausea.

Hemorrhoids are often caused by weak Spleen energy because weak Spleen energy can lead to a prolapse of the rectum, which is extremely painful. A good way to remedy this situation is to build up the Spleen energy. This can be done through acupressure, acupuncture, or a change of diet. Yams are very good for enhancing Spleen energy; four a day would be sufficient to have a beneficial effect on Spleen and thereby affect the hemorrhoids. But Western medicine would never associate Spleen with hemorrhoids, let alone yams, and would more than likely resort to surgery to fix the problem.

These are three simple examples of how pain makes little sense in terms of Western medicine yet, in each case, the problems are treatable by Oriental methods.

Make sure you chart pain in your daily listing of symptoms for self-diagnosis. Which flow passes through the area of pain?

Do you have different areas where pain occurs simultaneously? Which flows are involved? When does the pain occur; the Yin part of the day, or the Yang?

I know that for many of you, being asked to engage in self-diagnosis is a radical approach to illness and health. It is also the first stage in reclaiming your power over your own body and taking responsibility for your own well-being. As your skill in self-diagnosis improves, symptoms that seemed random and isolated will begin to form patterns.

Slowly, but surely, the pieces of the puzzle will begin to fall into place.

13

self-
awareness

BEING MINDFUL OF THE TRADITIONAL ASSOCIATIONS OF THE Five Elements in your daily living is important for charting what is really going on within your system. When imbalance exists—either excessive or depleted energy—paying attention to your body, and to tastes, smells, emotions, foods, herbs, and spices will help you on your quest for freedom from ill health. By looking at the lists on pages 63-65, Traditional Associations of the Five Elements, you will know which foods can help a particular organ pair become healthy, and which foods to refrain from eating if there is organ imbalance of an excessive type.

It is also important to chart the moon phases when figuring your natural pattern. Since each of the Five Elements is governed by a moon phase, and we see the moon most nights (depending what phase it is in), pay attention to its phases. How do you feel on a full moon? The full moon governs the Fire organs, which give energy to the Earth organs, which control the Water organs. Do you crave rice or apples or chicken or dates? Does your mouth have a bitter taste? Is there a putrid smell to your natural body odor? Do you feel like hibernating? Are you fearful around the time of the new moon? In this example, the foods, taste, odor, and behavior are all associated with the Water element organs. What shape is your Kidney flow in? It might be a good idea to wear some dark blue or black to help you through this moon phase and help your energy flows.

Are you having problems with your Liver? Old excessive anger on the rise? Well, go out in the desert or up in the mountains, anywhere you can be alone; roll up the windows in your car and *shout* during Liver's peak hours between 1-3 A.M. or low times from 1-3 P.M.

Trouble with your Heart? *Laugh* between 11-1 P.M. or 11-1 A.M. Troubles with your Earth organs, your Spleen or Stomach, your immune system? Then *sing* between 9-11 A.M. and 9-11 P.M., or in the shower between 7-9 A.M. or 7-9 P.M. The action of sound traveling through, into, and out of the body has a great healing effect.

Yogis don't chant for the fun of it or because they have nothing better to do with their time. They chant because chanting certain sounds (such as OM or A-E-I-O-U vowel chants— in as low a tone as possible) raises their inner vibrations to a higher spiritual level. Have you ever been to a rock concert where the music was so loud you felt it bouncing around inside you, and your body started to buzz or pound and pulsate internally with the drum as the drummer pounded out the beat? Read the information in Traditional Association, pages 63-65. Absorb the information into your subconscious, and into your intuition, and apply the knowledge to all aspects of your everyday living. Shout, sing, laugh, groan, weep, or wail your way to health and clear out unwanted "bad" stored organ energy!

Be your own detective, your own cartographer, mapping imbalances in your body. Look at all the times you have been ill or undergone surgery. What organ was involved? Did the illness follow a traumatic event in your life? Which side of your body was involved? Which foot do you repeatedly bash into furniture? Which ankle do you sprain time and time again? What is your body trying to tell you? Is it saying, "Do I have to get this sick for you to notice what you are doing to yourself and me, your body?"

Keep a journal or notebook handy and begin to look at your whole life through Five Element eyes. Review the illnesses that you, your parents, or grandparents developed. What are your dreams trying to tell you about your present health or your ancestors' lives?

As soon as I understand something about myself—the roots of a destructive pattern perhaps—with that understanding comes my first step towards wholeness and health. Why, in the past, have I been attracted to men who ultimately betrayed me and with whom I experienced so much pain? What was that pain trying to tell me, and what was the origin of the pain in the first place? Was the pain left over from events in my childhood, or was it pain from a current situation? Why do I sometimes deny my intuition, my psyche, my knowing? When is patience no longer a virtue but harmful to one's own being?

In the depths of your mind is your Soul, and when your Soul understands, so does your brain. When your brain understands, then and only then, can it send out messages to the body to heal because it finally knows the root of the problem or illness.

PART THREE

The Twenty-Four Forbidden Pregnancy Points

14

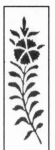 *a new perspective for women*

BY THIS POINT, A NEW PERSPECTIVE IS FORMING: YOU WILL HAVE begun to see that the body is an interconnected system of energies acting, interacting, and reacting; and that body, mind, and spirit come together and unite to form the whole woman. We can now begin to understand that the body's energy is fluid and everchanging, that the energy flows of the body are in a constantly fluctuating state of cause and effect, action and reaction, and have an internal clock all of their own. Everything that affects us—from the food we eat, to stress on the job—is taken in and processed by our internal organs and energy flows. This holistic concept—that there is a constant interchange of energy flow between the body, mind, and emotions—is the key to working with the Forbidden Pregnancy Points System presented in this section.

Because menstruation is a unique and special aspect of being female, most women know—if not in our minds, at least intuitively, in our gut—that the body, the mind, and the emotions are all interrelated. Cramping, sleeplessness, fatigue, heaviness, dizziness, nausea, backache, bloating, irritablity, depression—we've come to expect some or all of these every twenty-eight days. No wonder many women refer to their periods as the Curse. How wide a range these symptoms cover!

My intention in writing this book is to provide women with a simple and effective means for healing gynecological problems. The Forbidden Pregnancy Points System is based upon my study of the twenty-four Forbidden Pregnancy Points of Oriental medicine, as well as my practical experience as an acupressure and auricular therapist already working with the traditional points through acupressure. In my quest to learn more about the points, I had stubbornly persisted until I finally found the answer to my original question, "When do we work these points?" The answer is: *When we menstruate.*

These Forbidden Points, which can have such a powerful and harmful effect on pregnancy, can have an equally powerful—and beneficial—effect when used during the menstrual cycle. During this time, the power of the points can be used to pull energy out of the body, to work with the natural cycle of menstruation to shed old energy, energy that leaves the body as menstrual blood.

By working with the points during menstruation on a regular basis, this pulling out of old energy also strengthens and increases the longevity of our reproductive systems, therefore keeping menopause and menopause symptoms at bay a little longer.

Using this System, I have freed myself of awful gynecological problems, which had spanned twenty-five years, including chronic endometriosis. I found that the Forbidden Points could be used to relieve PMS, and to alleviate cramps and an overly-heavy menstrual flow. What's more, the points can be used to regulate the onset of menstruation and ovulation. During my investigation into the effective use of the points, I developed a contraceptive system that actually worked for me; a system, moreover, that guaranteed me my period with predictable regularity each month.

Friends and clients with whom I have shared this massage technique have reported results similar to my own, with PMS, cramps, and long periods being eliminated from their monthly cycles. I came to think of the Forbidden Points as feminine *empowerment* points. For the 90s "empowerment" is a bit passé; the word really sprang to life in the 80s, and yet it's what sprang to mind. The proper use of these points really does give us power over the female body. When we can control our own monthly cycles, which are at the very core of our femaleness, we are truly in control of our bodies, and our lives.

Woman Heal Thyself was written to present you with the Forbidden Pregnancy Points System, a system developed to balance your menstrual cycle at its most fundamental level. In this section, we will look at three specific uses of the System:

• How to regulate your menstrual cycle each month to rid yourself of the primary imbalance at the root of your menstrual problems, which are the cause of symptoms of PMS (chapter 16).

• Once mastered, how to use the System to actually bring on your period every month, a technique that can serve as a gentle and noninvasive form of birth control, or because you have reason to believe your period won't come (chapter 17).

• How the System can work to stave off the onset of menopause through its flushing out qualities (chapter 18).

The array of problems that can manifest gynecologically is vast. Premenstrual syndrome, or PMS, is a broad term, which, in addition to cramping, backache, and physical pain, can encompass the following:[1]

• Anxiety, irritability, mood swings, tension—shared by 70 percent of PMS sufferers;

• Bloating, fluid retention, weight gain, breast tenderness—shared by 60 percent;

1. Denise Foley and Eileen Nechas, *Women's Encyclopedia of Health and Emotional Healing* (Emmaus, PA: Rodale Press, 1993), p. 384.

• Cravings for sweets, dizziness, fatigue, headache, increased appetite, palpitations—symptoms shared by 30 to 40 percent of women;

• Confusion, crying, depression, forgetfulness, insomnia, withdrawal—shared by up to 20 percent of PMS sufferers.

You may suffer from one or all or many of these symptoms—or from others not even listed here. You should be aware that the System presented in this book is designed to balance and regulate the menses, and thereby bring harmony to the whole body. You cannot pick up this book on a Monday, and on Tuesday press a Forbidden Point to clear up "PMS"—whatever that might mean for you. Although we all share the same fundamental traits and biology, each woman has her own PMS to deal with. Where one woman might suffer largely from bloating and edema, another woman will experience PMS as constipation, and depression. Over time, through self-awareness and self-massage, you will come to know your own system. You will begin to notice relief of your symptoms, and a gentler period overall.

Because each woman is unique, I have also included in Part Five of this book a Diagnostic Reference list for those who wish to look up additional specific acupressure points for certain ailments that can accompany menstruation—such as acne, breast pain, depression, and so on. The Diagnostic Reference list will also address particular concerns not covered in this section, such as postpartum recovery, help during the birthing process, breast-feeding and weaning.

Although I am not an M.D., I have passed on what I have learned to many women. I have seen a career woman reverse menopause, which had set in when she was thirty-five, so that at forty-two years of age she could realistically think about having children when the "right" man appeared in her life. Another client of mine began using the System, rid herself of endometriosis, conceived and gave birth to a healthy baby girl, all in the space of one year. Three desperate friends, one of whom had been raped, terminated pregnancies within the first trimester of those pregnancies, simply by massaging certain areas of their bodies.

My original focus for this work was healing my own gynecological problems. I did not research the Forbidden Points in order to terminate pregnancies, although it must be restated and made clear that these twenty-four points have been "Forbidden" for so long precisely *because* of their power to terminate a pregnancy. In the acupressure charts that follow on pages 118 through 131, I have clearly indicated each point, its location, and the month from which it should not be worked if you are pregnant and wish to remain so.

But what if we could control our own cycles so that our periods could arrive on a regular schedule, and arrive gently? What if we could control our cycles so that we are no longer bothered by menopause? What if we could manage our cycles so that we would be assured of a period every month; so that we could decide when, and if, we want to conceive? Well, we can.

The Forbidden Pregnancy Points System can be used as a method of birth control. Although this technique took me months to master, it came about as a by-product of healing other gynecological problems, and by religiously practicing the System I developed for myself when my bleeding naturally began. It was only later in my research, after I had started to explore what I could do for myself in terms of contraception by means of energy management, that I learned to bring on my own period each month. This System is shared with you in chapter 17, "How to Bring On Your Period."

You must become totally familiar with your body's energy flows, and master the system of regulation presented in chapter 16, before you can learn the contraceptive method. For that reason, this book is primarily about learning to heal yourself of menstrual cycle problems. *Note well*: Some people may never be able to regulate their energy to the point that they can effectively bring on their own period, while others may do so very easily. You will need to be rigorously honest with yourself. If you are still experiencing PMS and other menstrual problems, *it is too soon to employ the contraceptive method yourself.* However, a competent and willing acupuncturist or acupressurist could administer this monthly "bring-on-the-period" method for you.

We must learn to walk before we can run. And yet, Oriental medicine is so all-encompassing and user-friendly that you will learn to run extremely well if you apply yourself.

15

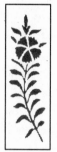

method for
working
the points

THE METHOD FOR MASSAGING THE POINTS IS EASY. HOWEVER, it is important to remember that this System evolved over time as a result of experimentation. First I had to understand the fundamentals of Oriental medicine and how illness occurs. Then I had to work with the twenty-four Forbidden Pregnancy Points and become familiar with a body, *my* body, which on some levels I was out of touch with, literally *out-of-touch* with. Then I had to chart the different changes within my body as I became familiar with that body. Through patience and discipline, this method took shape.

It was never a case of "Oh well, maybe I'll press a few points this month and maybe I won't." It was just the opposite. It was methodical; it took commitment and it took time. Time is one of the things most of us wish we had more of. How much do you hate PMS, or cramps or endless days of heavy bleeding? Are you willing to make the time to massage certain points on your body, without fail, every month when you bleed, each day of your period?

If you are willing to give yourself "me time" quite religiously, regularly, then you will have the chance to change aspects of your monthly cycle that you may well dread; unwanted aspects that my friends and clients also overcame because they were determined to take control of the only body they have. As the changes occur, one by one, you will know that you are mastering the System for regulating your menstrual cycle.

Once you can say to yourself, "I have no more PMS, or cramps, and my bleeding lasts for three days and is finished on the fourth"—then you know you are working successfully with your own energy.

A warning however: In one or two contemporary books that have been on the market for several years now, numerous Forbidden Pregnancy Points are listed throughout. One of these books in particular mentions the points with no word of caution in regards to pregnancy. I shudder to think how many women have followed exercise routines, pressed Forbidden Points while pregnant, and had miscarriages, never knowing why.

As I've said, it is my belief that the Forbidden Points hold a great deal of power. It is better that we understand them, and understand when and how to use them for our health, rather than just leave them lumped under the heading of "forbidden." *It is crucial for you to know not to stimulate them when you are pregnant.* It is just as important to know how to use them when you are not pregnant. I believe that by working these points we will stay younger for a longer period of time, menopause may well be delayed or reversed, and that great regenerative capabilities become available to us within their use.

This book, this System, is a way to understand yourself through Oriental medicine and, in the process of that understanding, come to know your own body. You will find that you will ask yourself "Which points were sore last month?" "Which points need the most attention this month?" But these are questions that you will ask with your hands, eventually without much conscious effort or thought. Making this System work depends on you. No one else. Give yourself permission to be self-centered; take time for yourself. Look over the last month. What happened in terms of your emotions and your life? Regret, sorrow, fear, the bad-credit blues? Match the emotions you experienced the most to the organ flows associated to those emotions, and then notice which points are the most sensitive.

Method for Massaging the Points*

SO HOW DO you begin? Before embarking on the Forbidden Pregnancy Points System outlined in chapter 16, you must be able to find your acupressure points! Pages 118 through 131 present the twenty-four Forbidden Pregnancy Points as they relate to the energy flows. Find the points on the body charts. Now locate that area on your own body.

Finding an acupressure point is a lot like finding the reflex point in your knee. You are shown where it is. You try tapping your knee a few times. Suddenly, when you do hit it, something quite beyond your control happens: your knee jerks. Locating that point again becomes easier and easier, and finally automatic as the memory gets stored in your body and your mind.

On your first look for your acupressure points, you will have that same hunt and peck feeling. When you do press the point, you should be able to feel some pain or discomfort. You have located the point. If, however, you locate the point area but have no real sensation there, you may have an energetic block, or an energetic gap between points. Knowing that there is a blockage won't be always obvious to you.

Using the Forbidden Pregnancy Points System does not require special clothing, a meditative posture, or special lighting. Working these points is something you can do at home, or at the office, or on the bus—anywhere that you feel comfortable massaging your ankles, knees, feet, forearm, and so on. I have listed beneficial time slots for working each of the points

*The Forbidden Pregnancy Points should *not* be worked on non-menstruating girls. Their bodies are still developing, and developing at their own pace, and should not be meddled with.

so that you can take advantage of the greatest energy the point has to offer. And yet working the points during their peak time isn't essential. If necessary, you can work the points through your clothing (but *not* working through a barrier is preferred).

Your intuitive or gut feeling will tell you which direction—clockwise or counterclockwise—to massage the point, whether you have pain or not. Eventually, conscious thought won't even come into it. However, here are important guidelines for understanding the directional flow of energy through the body, in terms of Yin and Yang—left or right, inside or outside, up or down.

YIN
From inside to outside
From bottom to top
From right to left

YANG
From outside to inside
From top to bottom
From left to right

To Tonify or draw energy into the body, massage a point in a clockwise direction. To Sedate or reduce energy in the body, massage counterclockwise. This is a rule of Traditional Oriental Medicine. However, with regard to energy, we have to take into consideration what is said in the *Nan Jing—A Classic of Difficult Questions*—where it states:

Left corresponds to Emptiness while
Right corresponds to Fullness.

So here you must pay attention to which side of the body you are working with, left or right. To facilitate faster drainage of old energy, it sometimes helps to work the left side of the body more than the right. Or, if you prefer, simply press the area until the discomfort diminishes.

There is another consideration—the time of day. We know that organs have peak and low times of the day. It is always preferable to tonify an organ during its peak time slot, however this can become inconvenient when dealing with those flows that peak during the night. I personally do not get up between 3 and 5 A.M. to work my Lung points.

Everyone is different and that's the rule of thumb. Some months you may find yourself pressing the points, another month you will begin by massaging them in a counterclockwise direction to get rid of old energy, and finish by using the clockwise method to draw in new energy.

With your own two hands you will get in touch with your body as never before. You may even be able to feel your own energy gently pulsing beneath your fingers as it releases. If you don't feel a pulsing sensation, it doesn't matter—you will still achieve the same results. Or take this book to your massage therapist and have the therapist give you a good working over on these points. Let it become your once-a-month treat to yourself if you can afford it. Or have a friend help you with the System. Build a network of women who get together and help each other clear out these points each month. Perhaps your husband or partner would help massage the points—a pleasant way to connect in an intimate way at a time of the month when men often feel left out, ignored, and sexually frustrated.

That's it. Nothing mystical or complicated. The plain fact is that "the plain facts" have been kept from us, either by intention or by neglect, since ancient times. We could look on this withholding as a conspiracy to keep women in their place. Then again, perhaps it was not until now that we were ready to embrace and integrate this knowledge into our lives in a wise and meaningful way.

Let's start by looking at the locations of the twenty-four points, and the forbidden months during pregnancy. Pages 118 through 131 illustrate these twenty-four points by energy flow name. The points are circled, and are found in both right and left limbs, even though only one side may be shown.

Spleen Energy Flow

Point Number	Oriental Name	Forbidden From Month:
1	Hidden White	1
2	Great Capital	1
6	Three Yin Crossing	9

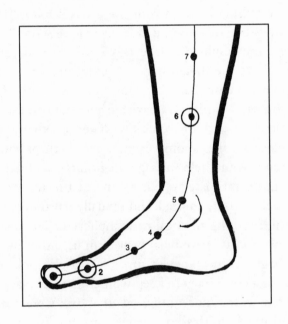

Stomach Energy Flow

POINT NUMBER	ORIENTAL NAME	FORBIDDEN FROM MONTH:
4	Earth Granary	5
36	Leg Three Miles	8
45	Severe Mouth	6

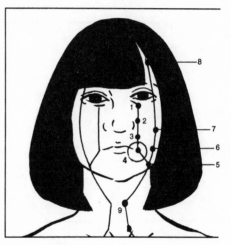

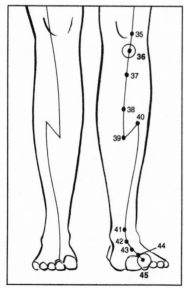

Lung Energy Flow

POINT NUMBER	ORIENTAL NAME	FORBIDDEN FROM MONTH:
7	Broken Sequence	6
11	Little Merchant	7

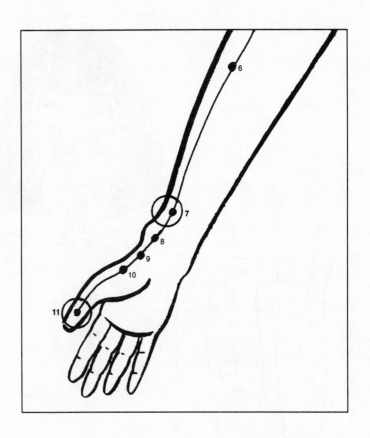

Large Intestine Energy Flow

POINT NUMBER	ORIENTAL NAME	FORBIDDEN FROM MONTH:
2	Second Space	9
4	Ho Ku or Tiger's Mouth or Joining The Valleys or Great Eliminator	1-9
10	Arm Three Miles	9

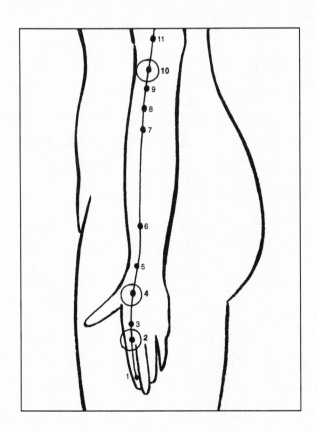

Kidney Energy Flow

POINT NUMBER	ORIENTAL NAME	FORBIDDEN FROM MONTH:
1	Bubbling Spring	1 & 8
2	Blazing Valley or Dragon in the Abyss/Spring	8
4	Great Bell	3
7	Returning Flow	8

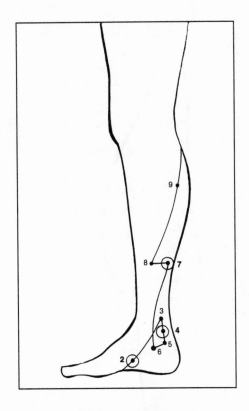

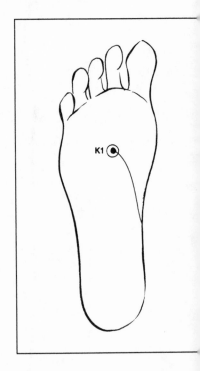

Gallbladder Energy Flow

POINT NUMBER	ORIENTAL NAME	FORBIDDEN FROM MONTH:
2	Hearing Assembly	1
9	Heaven Rushing	4
34	Yang Mound Spring	2

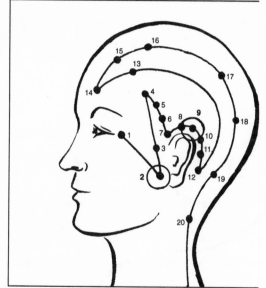

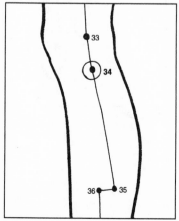

Small Intestine Energy Flow

Point Number	Oriental Name	Forbidden From Month:
7	Regulating Branch or Branch to the Correct	6
10	Shoulder Blade	6

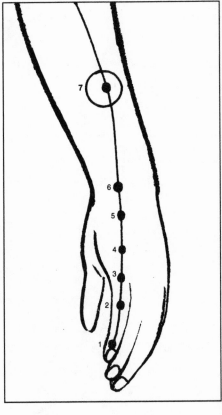

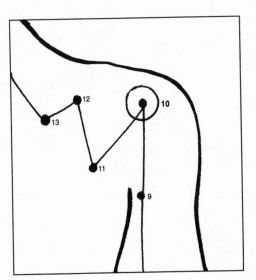

Pericardium Energy Flow

POINT NUMBER	ORIENTAL NAME	FORBIDDEN FROM MONTH:
6	Inner Frontier Gate	4
8	Palace of Weariness	3

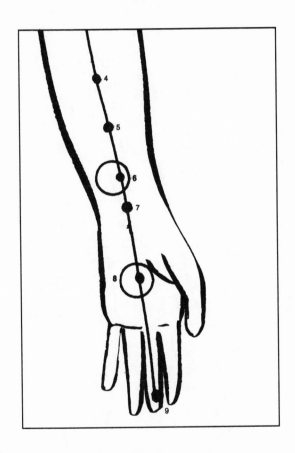

Triple Warmer Energy Flow

POINT NUMBER	ORIENTAL NAME	FORBIDDEN FROM MONTH:
4	Yang Pond	3
10	Heavenly Well	3-5

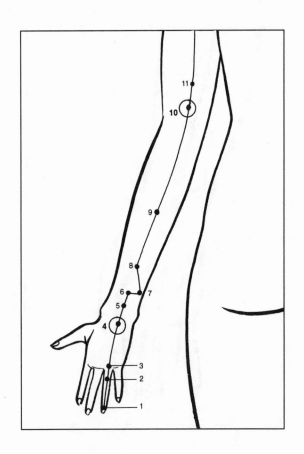

Additional Points

The following additional points are not traditionally given the name of Forbidden Pregnancy Points, like the twenty-four we have just looked at. However, I am including them because they have been known to have an adverse effect on pregnancy, since they have a "clearing out" effect and relax the womb. They are also beneficial during menstruation for the following varied reasons:

Spleen 4 is helpful in relieving cramps; it causes the uterus to relax.

Spleen 9 is the Water Point of Spleen and helps to relieve swelling, edema (water retention), and generally has a regulating effect on Spleen.

Kidney 6 has a strengthening effect on the uterus and is good for prolapse. It also helps relieve cramps, swelling, and helps to clear up irregular menstruation.

Liver 3 is known for opening the womb (dilating the cervix). It helps with edema and relieves constipation, which can cause "pressure pains" against the uterus.

Gallbladder 41 serves to eliminate pain and swelling in the breasts and to reduce abdominal distention. A good working of this point will, over time, help stop the premenstrual pain, tenderness, and swelling of the breasts in your next cycle.

It is important to be aware of the potential power of all points, not just those called "forbidden." They are included in the System that I'm presenting here because they are beneficial in treating menstrual problems because of their "flushing out" and balancing properties.

These additional points have been boxed for easy identification. The flows are found on both arms and legs, even though only one may be shown.

Spleen Energy Flow

POINT NUMBER	ORIENTAL NAME
4	Prince's Grandson
9	Yin Mound Spring

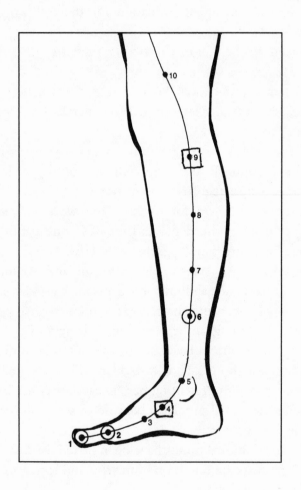

Kidney Energy Flow

POINT NUMBER   ORIENTAL NAME

6   Shining Sea

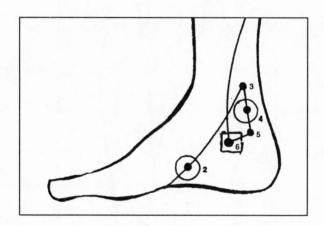

Liver Energy Flow

POINT NUMBER	ORIENTAL NAME
3	Supreme Rushing or Great Pouring

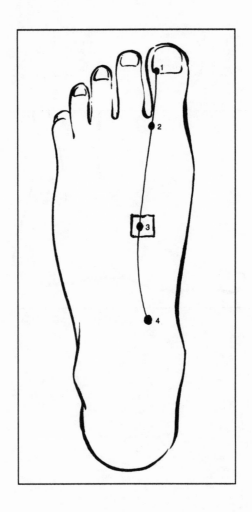

Gallbladder Energy Flow

POINT NUMBER   ORIENTAL NAME

41   Foot Overlooking Tears

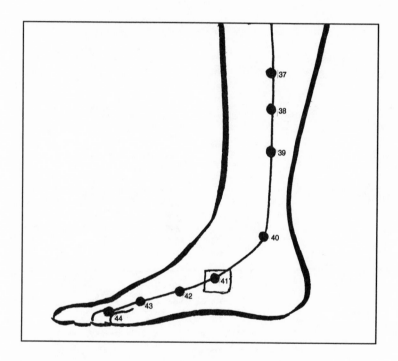

16

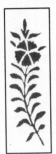

regulating
the menstrual
cycle

THE FORBIDDEN PREGNANCY POINTS SYSTEM USES THE POWER
of the Forbidden Points in a healing, beneficial way. While you
are menstruating, you will work with the flow of the energy in
your body.

What does this method do? It balances your body energy
at a very fundamental level so that total harmony is achieved.
An ambitious claim! But as you become more self-aware, and
more acquainted with the concept of Yin and Yang and the patterns of interchange among the Five Elements; as you become
more conscious of what goes on in that body of yours on a daily
basis—physically, emotionally, spiritually—you will begin to
understand that pain, discomfort, and irritability are never the
body's normal state of balance.

On the first day of your period, massage the points in the
order listed on pages 136 through 138, and continue until the
bleeding cycle has finished. I have presented four sets of points
to correspond with the average number of days a woman has
her period. If your cycle is only three days, then end with the
third set. If your bleeding continues into days five, six, or seven,
you start again with set one and repeat the sets in order until

the bleeding stops. What I have found with most women is that, after using this System, the cycle balances out to four days.

NOTE: The bold headings at the top of each set reference the months during which these points are forbidden when you are pregnant.

During your period, the points should be massaged at least once a day, each for about two to five minutes. I generally massage them as close to their peak time slot as possible, but tend to do a morning group and then an evening group. The Ho Ku Points (Large Intestine 4) can be massaged many times throughout the day. These points are so powerful that the time of day they are worked really has little to do with it.

Remember, counterclockwise will disperse old energy and clockwise will bring in new energy. Always massage in a clockwise direction on the last day of your period to make sure you have drawn in a good supply of fresh energy.

If you get confused about which direction is clockwise, your head is the number 12 position on the clock, and the "face" would be the front of your body, so your left arm would be where the number 3 position is and you right arm, the number 9 position. No matter which side of your body, arm, or leg you are working, the "view" is always as if you were looking at yourself.

I have indicated that you should work each point from two to five minutes. After a while, you will discover the length of time that works best for you—it could be longer or shorter. The length of time spent massaging the point will vary from individual to individual. Some people release energy more slowly, others more quickly. Then again, some points are more powerful than others, and require pressure, but less time. When you're comfortable with the basics of massaging each point, go to chapter 25, "Ancient Point Use Rules," where you will find more advanced instruction for working with the specific energy of different points.

The points listed in brackets in "Set 1" are the additional points—not Forbidden—that I also work every month, because they have a clearing out effect.

Keep in mind:
- The points should be worked in the order listed
- Counterclockwise flushes out old energy
- Clockwise brings in fresh energy
- Work each point from two to five minutes

Day 1 of Period Work Set #1
Day 2 of Period Work Set #2
Day 3 of Period Work Set #3
Day 4 of Period Work Set #1

SET ONE

One to Three Months

Flow	Point	Peak Time
LARGE INTESTINE	4	5-7 A.M.
SPLEEN	1, 2, (4, 9)	9-11 A.M.
KIDNEY	1, 4, (6)	5-7 P.M.
PERICARDIUM	8	7-9 P.M.
TRIPLE WARMER	4, 10	9-11 P.M.
GALLBLADDER	2, 34, (41)	11 P.M.-1 A.M.
LIVER	(3)	1-3 A.M.

SET TWO

Three to Six Months

Flow	Point	Peak Time
LUNG	7	3-5 A.M.
LARGE INTESTINE	4	5-7 A.M.
STOMACH	4, 45	7-9 A.M.
SMALL INTESTINE	7, 10	1-3 P.M.
KIDNEY	4	5-7 P.M.
PERICARDIUM	6	7-9 P.M.
TRIPLE WARMER	10	9-11 P.M.
GALLBLADDER	9	11 P.M.-1 A.M.

SET THREE

Six to Nine Months

Flow	Point	Peak Time
LUNG	11	3–5 A.M.
LARGE INTESTINE	2, 4, 10	5–7 A.M.
STOMACH	36	7–9 A.M.
SPLEEN	6	9–11 A.M.
KIDNEY	1, 2, 7	5–7 P.M.

Short Version of the Monthly Clear Out

The points listed below are the original set that I worked on myself, without fail, every month for six months. By the third month, I had no more PMS problems or troubles with my period. For the rest of that first year, I continued putting together the other sequences, which I worked for another full year and still do today. These sets also contain the Additional Points, shown in boxes on pages 128 through 131.

Flow	Point	Peak Time
SPLEEN	1, 2, 4, 6, 9	9–11 A.M.
STOMACH	36	7–9 A.M.
LARGE INTESTINE	4	5–7 A.M.
KIDNEY	1, 6	5–7 P.M.
GALLBLADDER	41	11 P.M.–1 A.M.

This one set of points is worked every day of your period until the bleeding stops.

The Short Version is for women who, for one reason or another, simply cannot fit the three sets of points into their lives. Some people dislike following any type of regimen, while others seem too busy or scattered to try anything that has more than one step to it. So, if you have time to work only two of these points a few times a day while your period is in progress, let those points be Large Intestine 4 and Spleen 6 (see pages 121 and 118). These two points are the most powerful of all the Forbidden Pregnancy Points. However, by working *all* the points mentioned in the previous chapter, broader balancing occurs, and helps to regulate mid-month ovulation. This is a relatively simple method for balancing your whole female system, from the beginning of a monthly cycle (menstruation), straight through to the next cycle.

Results

You will know that you have begun to achieve the positive effects of this System when your PMS symptoms vanish. Generally, swelling will go first, then cramping. You know what your problems are, so when you begin the System, write them down in list form. For example:

Week prior to period
Legs swollen, breasts sore and swollen. Crabby, snappish, weepy, insecure . . .
Bleeding days:
Bleeding very heavy, terrible cramps, nauseated first day. Second day still heavy bleeding, cramps so bad I can't think straight . . .

Friends and clients alike have benefited from doing this simple monthly routine, reporting that they feel better, their problems have cleared up, and they look younger as a result.

17

how to
bring on
your period

FOR THOSE OF YOU WHO HAVE ELIMINATED ALL MENSTRUAL
cycle problems using the Forbidden Pregnancy Points System
outlined in this book, this contraceptive method is also included for your use. In undertaking this method of contraception,
you do so at your own risk. The risk? An unwanted pregnancy
if you fail to succeed in mastering this more advanced stage of
regulating your own energy.

Let's say you know the length of your monthly cycle—
twenty-eight, twenty-nine, or thirty days—so you can predict
with considerable accuracy when your period is due. Suppose
your period is due on day twenty-eight. Using a twenty-
eight-day cycle as an example, this is what you do. On day
twenty-five—the third day prior to the due date—start using
the Short Version of the System outlined in chapter 16, massaging the most powerful of the Forbidden Points beginning
at 9-11 A.M., the peak hours for Spleen Flow in the twenty-
four-hour cycle. The routine would go as follows:

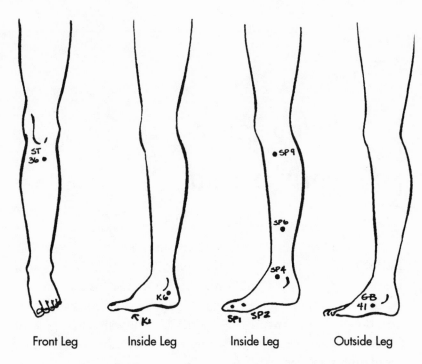

Front Leg   Inside Leg   Inside Leg   Outside Leg

SP = Spleen; ST = Stomach; LI = Large Intestine; K = Kidney; GB = Gallbladder

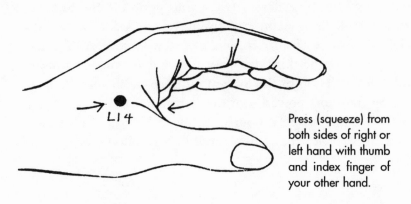

Press (squeeze) from both sides of right or left hand with thumb and index finger of your other hand.

DAY 25:

Flow	Point	Peak/Low Time
SPLEEN	1, 2, 4, 6, 9	9-11 A.M./P.M.
STOMACH	36	7-9 A.M./P.M.
LARGE INTESTINE	4	5-7 A.M./P.M.
KIDNEY	1, 6	5-7 P.M./A.M.
GALLBLADDER	41	11 P.M./A.M.–1 A.M./P.M.

All of these points, with the exception of Ho Ku, Large Intestine 4, are found on your lower leg, from the knee to the ball of the foot. If you happen to be at work on day twenty-five, concentrate on working the less obvious flows, such as Large Intestine 4. At the end of the day, when you get home, finish with the Spleen, Stomach, Kidney, and Gallbladder Flow points. Pay attention to the low hours between 9-11 P.M. for Spleen. Why? The object of this technique is to disperse energy massaging the points in a *counterclockwise* direction. During the low hours, a flow is at its most vulnerable, and you can easily disperse *more* energy by working the points during this time.

Continue this point massage on days twenty-six, twenty-seven, and twenty-eight, by which time you will have brought on your bleeding.

Or, your acupuncturist can work these points for you, as described in *Acupuncture: A Comprehensive Text:*[1]

> Needle Large Intestine 4 with mild stimulation. Needle Spleen 6 with strong stimulation, directing the needle upwards so that the sensation extends to the lower abdomen. Use slanted insertion at Governing Vessel 1 to a depth of approximately 3 units. Direct the needle upward at this point so that the sensation extends to the lumbosacral region. The needle at Spleen 9

1 John O'Connor and Dan Bensky, Shanghai College of Traditional Medicine, *Acupuncture: A Comprehensive Text*, Sixth Edition (Seattle: Eastland Press, 1988), p. 678.

should also be directed upwards so that the sensation reaches the inguinal canal. The two principal (L14 and SP6) and supplementary (GV1 and SP9) points should be used in rotation. Treat once daily for 2-3 consecutive days.

Remember to think about what you are doing in terms of Oriental medicine, and what has been discussed in previous chapters. It's important that you understand Five Element theory, so that you will be aware of the interrelatedness of all parts of your body, your mind, and your spirit. Be mindful that Spleen governs the sexual energy, that Stomach is Spleen's partner, and that Kidney stores sexual energy. Large Intestine is the "child" of Stomach and therefore is capable of taking energy away.

Stomach 36 and 45 are both powerful dispersion points, as are Kidney 1, Triple Warmer 10, Large Intestine 2, 4, and 10. It is possible to regulate Stomach, Spleen, and Kidney flows from Stomach 36, and Stomach 45 flows into the Spleen flow at Spleen 1. Pay particular attention to these points and massage them collectively for twenty minutes, three times a day.

Once you have brought on your period, continue to use the System just as if your period had occurred naturally. This is how you regulate your body function harmoniously and with grace. Once a month, time is spent massaging the Forbidden Points, and this practice regulates the next cycle. Time, diligence, patience, and intention go a long way here.

This method of bringing on your period assumes that (1) you have reason to believe that you may have conceived and your period will not arrive as due; or (2) you are relying on this system as your method of contraception.

Taoist Secrets Hidden in Poetry

Much can be learned from paying attention to Chinese point names, poetry, and legends which often have profound or double meanings. Sometimes information is disguised and hidden within the lines of simple story or rhyme. In this way a master's healing secrets were kept hidden and passed only from teacher to student. The actual Chinese character (letter) for "acupuncture point" means hole or cave.

I have read many Chinese poems, translated from the original texts by Westerners, and I know that these poems contain clues and instructions relating to certain acupressure points and their effect upon the female body. It is sad that the majority of these texts have been translated by individuals who have demonstrated little knowledge of Oriental medicine and point names. So once again, this time through poor translation, we are losing vital information pertinent to women.

However, if you wish to read beautiful examples of well translated works written by women and relating to women, then reach for Thomas Cleary's wonderful book, *Immortal Sisters: Secrets of Taoist Women*. For example, here is a poem by Zhou Xuanjing. Listen with different ears, and see with different eyes.

> *Essence and life must first be studied*
> *In the moon cave;*
> *Capture the dragon, bind the tiger*
> *Do not delay.*
> *If yang leaks out during its development,*
> *How can the granule be preserved whole?* [2]

To me, this classical poem relates to life, the feminine, to energy, and gestation; it refers to specific points and, as is the case with many Taoist writings, when we read between the lines, another level of information can be discovered.

Moon is associated with Yin, Cave is another name for point, but Moon Cave is also a colloquial expression for the womb or the vagina. The Dragon is associated with fertility, and

2. Thomas Cleary, *Immortal Sisters: Secrets of Taoist Women* (Boston: Shambhala, 1989), p. 83. Reprinted by permission.

in essence to "capture the Dragon" would be to control fertility. To "bind the Tiger" could refer to either Governing Vessel 1 or Large Intestine 4 in terms of arresting and dispersing the energy at those points, since both points are associated with contraception or therapeutic abortion. "Granule" could reference a seed of life in a woman's belly; with leaking Yang energy, its development could be impaired.

Governing Vessel 1, most commonly called Long Strong—a reference to the penis, due to its location at the base of the spine between the legs and the fact that it is a Yang energy flow—is also known as Dragon Tiger or Dragon and Tiger Point.

In ancient legends, the Tiger was associated with Yin, the female, the West and also with death. Tiger Step is one of the thirty traditional positions for lovemaking. The Dragon was associated with the East and fertility. Large Intestine 4 is also known as Tiger's Mouth.

Another point generally associated with miscarriage is Bladder 67, which is named Reaching Yin. It is the final point of the Bladder energy flow, a Yang flow. At this point Bladder passes energy along to its Yin partner, Kidney. By massaging Bladder 67 and Kidney 1—a Forbidden Point—what are you doing? You are dispersing energy from both flows.

The Immortal Sisters, all of them, were Taoist Masters. It is said that they could move energy throughout their bodies by just thinking about it, focusing the mind, seeing the energy move, in out up down, and it was so. I have been practicing meditation all my life, and as of the writing of this book, I still have problems moving energy "just" by thinking about it. This is a way of life, not a health fad of the moment.

I encourage you to write me at the address at the back of this book with any difficulties or questions and to share with me your experiences in using the System.

18

pre-menopause and menopause

USUALLY AFTER THE AGE OF FORTY, ALTHOUGH SOMETIMES earlier, a woman will enter a pre-menopausal state. This stage of a woman's life may last anywhere from two to ten years and will be different for every woman.

During pre-menopause, a woman's body undergoes changes that can be quite confusing, debilitating, and alarming. The ovaries gradually stop producing the female hormone estrogen in the amounts that our bodies are accustomed to during most of our adult life. This occurs prior to menopause when estrogen levels actually peak, and progesterone production declines. At this stage of pre-menopause, the most varied symptoms may be experienced. Then estrogen production declines even further, levels off, and yet the ovaries continue to make testosterone and androstenedione—two male hormones. Even when we are in our late seventies, small amounts of estrogen are still present in our bodies.

Often menstrual periods will become irregular—longer or shorter bleeding days, longer or shorter times between cycles, spotting at mid-month. Ovulation will be irregular, occurring at the end of a month, the beginning of the month, or not at all during some cycles.

There may be changes in skin texture with loss of elasticity and moisture content so that dryness and wrinkles become more prevalent. There may be a loss of interest in sex. Vaginal changes such as dryness and itchiness may occur, as well as urinary incontinence and bladder infections caused by decreased friendly flora in the vagina.

The lack of moisturizing secretions in the body can also extend to dryness of the nasal passages, throat, and upper lung area, and make you more susceptible to colds and coughs. Tear ducts become drier and may result in dry eyes. Problems wearing contact lenses may occur. Loss of elasticity in the skin results in breasts beginning to sag and shrink in size. The nipples may lose their capacity for sexual arousal and erectness. Hair may increase on the chest, stomach area and face. The voice may deepen. Muscle tone might be lost in the body overall. With muscle tone loss, the uterus can drop, become prolapsed. There may be a sensation of tingling under the skin and numbness in the hands, arms, and legs. Lumbar pain, mental instability, a ringing in the ears (tinnitus), or a tickling feeling as if tiny invisible insects are crawling across the skin—all of these are possible symptoms.

Eyesight may suddenly worsen or improve. Weight gain, palpitations of the heart, sluggish blood circulation, shortness of breath, or a feeling that the air is being sucked from a room may occur. Women experience depression, memory loss, panic attacks, headaches, sudden claustrophobia, paranoia, and sleepless nights. All of this from lack of estrogen!

Because estrogen is required for calcium assimilation, osteoporosis—weak and brittle bones—can become a problem as a result of a calcium deficiency. Calcium supplements, about 800mg, should be taken daily, along with 400 I.U. of vitamin D, which aids absorption of calcium. Smoking, alcohol, and caffeine inhibit the absorption of calcium. A balanced diet is essential in the pre-menopausal and menopausal phases of life, especially if you haven't paid much attention to a proper nutritious diet earlier in life.

Foods that are beneficial for pre- and menopausal women are the following: carrots, yams, brown rice, beans, miso, tofu, potatoes, peas, collard greens, broccoli, pink salmon, apples, sardines, sesame seeds, cod liver oil, eggs, tuna, soy foods, pumpkin seeds, buckwheat, cherries, grapes, citrus fruits. Avoid caffeine and too much salt.

Almost every woman's vote for the worst symptom of all is hot flashes. Hot flashes—a feeling that you are on fire while oozing buckets of water, with red splotches appearing on the face, neck, and upper chest—can occur day or night, last for varying lengths of time, and hit without warning. Pre-menopause can be living hell. Then again, you may be one of 15 percent of all women who enter this pre-menopausal stage completely without symptoms. If you are, congratulations!

Menopause Onset

At the time of this writing, thirteen million women in the United States alone are already in menopause. This figure does not include the baby-boomers, who are soon to join these ranks in large numbers.

The state of menopause is said to have been reached when a woman has missed twelve consecutive menstrual cycles; anything prior to this last missed menstrual period is pre-menopause.

Energetically, menopause begins because of weak and declining Kidney energy to the point of eventual emptiness. This depletion leads to emptiness of Heart and then Spleen, which leads to an imbalance of energy flow in the blood. If you look at all the relatively strange symptoms or side effects of pre-menopause you will see that they result from classic imbalances of Spleen, Kidney, and Heart (see pages 85 through 92, Physical Function of the Organs).

By keeping Kidney, Heart, and Spleen flows healthy in all

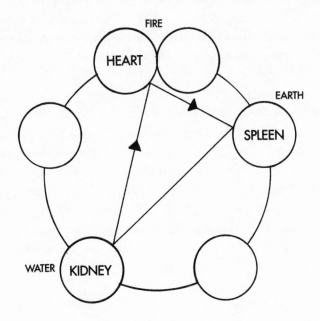

Energy depletion during menopause

aspects of daily living—free from emotional stress, nourished
with wholesome nutrition—menopause will come later in life,
when we desire it to happen. You may even find you can extend
your childbearing years.

Menopause will cease to be as difficult as our first menstruating years; it can be a time when our bodies will have settled into our own natural rhythm. Hormonal fluctuations will
be a thing of the past.

One client came to me seeking help with menopause. She
had entered menopause relatively early, at thirty-five years of
age. She was a dedicated career woman and, at the time, saw this
condition as more of a relief than a problem. When she was
forty-two, however, something quite unexpected happened. She
met a man who did more than just excite her about business

plans and ventures. Her interests began to include thoughts of marriage and family.

At our first meeting, she seemed desperate to change the state of her body. I taught her Five Element theory, and explained how energy depletion dominoes into physical symptoms. I taught her the Forbidden Pregnancy Points System, and she started using the method a few days prior to the next full moon. Because women in menopause are not menstruating, they obviously can't start when their periods begin! The full moon is the time of month that will traditionally give energy to the Fire organs, which then give energy to the Earth organs. Menopause occurs when Kidney (Water) energy becomes depleted, followed by Heart (Fire), and then Spleen (Earth), which governs the sexual organs.

She followed the system outlined in chapter 17, "How To Bring On Your Period," as if she were in a non-menopausal state. At the end of a week, she had her first bleeding in seven years. She continued to massage the points, and continued her therapy sessions during this time. Even though the romance did not blossom as she had hoped, she did get in touch with her body, her emotions, and her true feminine nature.

Pre-menopausal and menopausal women will benefit from tonifying the Forbidden Pregnancy Points once a month during the full moon—the moon phase that governs the Fire element. Also, massaging the following additional points helps Fire give energy to Spleen flow.

To tonify the Kidney, massage Kidney 3, 7, Bladder 23, 52, Conception Vessel 4.

To tonify the Heart, massage Heart 1, 7, Spleen 6, 9, Pericardium 6, 7, Conception Vessel 17.

To tonify the Spleen, massage Spleen 2, 3, Stomach 36, Bladder 20, Liver 13, and Conception Vessel 12.

• Work the points for four days beginning a few days prior to the full moon.

• Work the points in the order listed.

• Massage in a clockwise direction (remember, you are tonifying, drawing energy *in*).

Women who are pre-menopausal should begin this regimen when they begin to notice the symptoms as outlined in this chapter.

19

ho ku point for energy and stress reduction

IF I AM FEELING TIRED FROM OVERWORK I WILL LIE DOWN, AND gently clasp my fingers in the Ho Ku hands position shown on page 152. I place my left foot over my right foot—ball of my left foot touching the top of my right foot by the big toe—and breathe gently until I feel as if I have recharged my batteries. (See figure on following page.) By very lightly touching Ho Ku in an interlocking grasp you have created a closed energetic circuit at hands and feet. Even though Ho Ku is a Forbidden Point, this meditation does not alter or upset the monthly cycle in any way; it boosts the energy you have left in your body at the time.

The Ho Ku Revitalizing Exercise

This exercise is also very beneficial if you wake in the night and cannot get back to sleep. I have done this and found that although I may not have drifted off to sleep again right away, just doing this exercise revitalizes my mind and body, providing benefits similar to those of sleep.

Ho Ku-With-Feet is such a subtle exercise, that it can be done anywhere. Slip your shoes off, sit up straight, slip the left

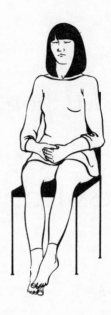

Posture for Ho Ku Meditation

foot over your right as illustrated here, and gently clasp your hands in your lap. Closing your eyes is not necessary, and you will enter a state of deep calm while remaining aware and clear-headed.

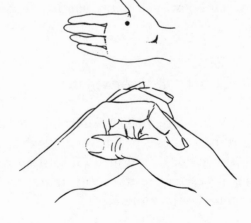

PART FOUR

Other Areas for Healing

20

the nature of disharmony, or why me?

IN THIS SECTION WE ARE GOING TO LOOK AT DEPRESSION, addiction, cervical cancer, sexually transmitted disease, and, in addition, address some problems that plague the men in our lives.

As with all the problems and conditions mentioned in this book, the following are serious, and you should not use this book to replace conventional medical treatment. Depression, panic attacks, addiction, compulsion, and cervical cancer are included here because research has shown a link between mind and body, and in many cases, such as depression, a significantly higher rate of illness occurs among women—in fact, twice as high: two women to every man. Why?

It has been shown that poor self-esteem has been linked to addiction, anorexia and bulimia, cervical cancer, and depression. Studies have found that 37 percent of all women suffering from depression had been sexually abused before the age of twenty-one. Roughly 30 percent to two-thirds of all women with eating disorders were sexually abused at some point in their lives. Forty percent of all American adults who abuse drugs and alcohol are women. Seventy percent of all women studied who were suffering from some form of addiction had been abused, either physically, sexually, or emotionally. A 1990 study found that 63 percent of all American women seeking outpatient psychiatric counseling, for a variety of reasons, were abused physically or sexually in childhood.[1]

In the Oriental holistic view, you cannot separate mind from body. As I mentioned earlier, many life experiences can manifest as dis-ease in other parts of the body, notably as gynecological problems. And stressors that affect the brain chemistry can start a chain reaction that can affect your body. Remember the theory of Yin and Yang—action and reaction, positive and negative. Your hormonal system is included in this cycle of interrelationship.

There is also a link between the body's hormones and diseases such as endometriosis. Endometriosis occurs when the endometrium starts to grow and attach itself *outside* the uterus in the abdominal cavity. The endometrium is the tissue that builds up and lines your womb in preparation for pregnancy. When you menstruate, you are shedding this lining. In the condition known as endometriosis, this lining literally backs up through the fallopian tubes and out of the uterus. It can attach itself to the ovaries, bladder, even the rectum. Once outside of the womb, the endometrium can play havoc with the abdominal organs as well.

Endometriosis can be an incredibly painful condition, one that many doctors are at a loss to explain, and that surgery does not always cure. There is not a lot of understanding as to why some women get it and some don't; there is speculation that it can be inherited genetically and is linked to the hormonal system. There is a Chinese herbal remedy called *Teng Long Tang*, or "Soaring Dragon Decoction," that is indicated in the treatment of endometriosis, as well as cervical and uterine

1. Denise Foley and Eileen Nechas, *Womens' Encyclopedia of Health and Emotional Healing* (Emmaus, PA: Rodale Press, 1993).pp. 130-132, 137, 162, 427.

cancers and tumors, and testitis in men. This treatment has been used successfully by Bob Flaws.[2]

Today an estimated 70 percent of women who suffer from endometriosis have probably been told by a doctor that the condition is psychological, or "in their heads." Eighty-three percent of women with endometriosis suffer severe pain throughout their cycle. Almost 20 percent of all hysterectomies performed are for the treatment of endometriosis.[3] Before I was cured, I ended up taking painkillers as extreme as codeine and morphine on a monthly basis.

When I started to work with my body's energy to address my gynecological problems, endometriosis was, I am grateful to report, one of the conditions that the Forbidden Points System addressed well. One of the clues for points therapy can be found in the description of endometriosis: in some cases the endometrium *backs up and out* of the fallopian tubes. This is energy moving in a Destructive Cycle. The regulating and balancing system presented in chapter 16 is working with a clockwise, Birthing Cycle, and will help you align your energy to flow in a balanced and healthy manner.

Finally, we will take a look at sexually transmitted disease. Did you know that for every woman with Chlamydia—the major cause of Pelvic Inflammatory Disease—there are 1.3 men who carry it? Did you know that of these women, 75 percent will show no symptoms?[4] In order to increase your awareness, we will make a brief overview of the illnesses that are out there, and discuss ways in which points can be used to boost your immune system.

There are several excellent books on the market that dis-

---

2. Bob Flaws, *Cervical Dysplasia & Prostate Cancer: HPV, A Hidden Link?* (Boulder, CO: Blue Poppy Press, 1990), page 177.
3. *Womens' Encyclopedia of Health and Emotional Healing,* pp. 164–167.
4. *ibid.,* pp. 440–441.

cuss these specific illnesses in depth, and several are listed in Recommended Reading at the back of the book.

Other ailments not covered in the section will be found in the Diagnostic Reference in Part Five.

21

 *depression and panic attacks*

DEPRESSION AND PANIC ATTACKS ARE FAR MORE SERIOUS THAN dark moods. Women who suffer from these illnesses are not being "emotional," an inaccurate cliché. We can't just be told to "pull ourselves up by our boot straps" (or sandal straps either). But we do have the capability of healing ourselves. By thinking positive thoughts we can learn to stop depression and panic attacks before they occur or take root. When we become depressed or begin to have a panic attack, a chemical imbalance actually occurs in the brain, and the situation goes from bad to worse to abject misery or terror.

A panic attack results from extreme anxiety and the reason for it is always personal to the individual experiencing it. An attack is usually caused by a fear or dread of a place or thing, perhaps elevators, or heights, airplanes, open spaces (including venturing outside the house), underground parking lots, nightmares, or a fearful thought that actually escalates within the imagination until it becomes out of control.

If you'd ever had a panic attack you'd know it! The fear is accompanied by physical sensations within the body, such as sweating, heart palpitations, trembling, a feeling that the chest is being pressed in upon so that breathing becomes near to impossible. Nausea and even diarrhea are present. Terror is all that exists.

The mind does a number on itself with fearful or imagined happenings; the thought process speeds up uncontrollably, goes into overdrive, and then outer orbit. The poor individuals going through this feel as though they'd like to crawl out of their skins and run away from the situation, away from their minds. Panic attacks have been known to lead to suicide because the terror is so enormous that some people can no longer bear what they are going through.

If we look at panic attacks in terms of Oriental Medicine and refer to "Anxiety" in the Diagnostic Reference, we see that the points that can be used for relief are the following: Stomach 36, Large Intestine 4, Kidney 1, Bladder 60, Liver 2, Heart 5 and 7, Small Intestine 4, and Pericardium 9. Please note that some are Forbidden Points.

In understanding why these points work we find the real clue to what is going on here: A panic attack really begins with the way the *mind* perceives *reality*. Chapter 11, which covers the physical function of the organs, also lists their Mental Function.

The Stomach is responsible for the digestion of thoughts; Large Intestine eliminates all impure thoughts; the Kidney deals with creating an open mind and clarity of thought; the Bladder eliminates impure ideas; the Liver gives strength to foresight and planning; the Heart coordinates all mental function; the Small Intestine discriminates between pure and impure (real and unreal) thoughts; and the Pericardium supports self-worth.

So in working with these points at the onset of a panic attack, you are going straight to fixing problems of mental function in the *mind*. During a panic attack, the panic of the mind has overloaded Stomach's ability to digest thoughts—physical nausea manifests. Large Intestine is attempting to remove all impure thoughts as fast as possible—excessive sweating. Kidney, overwhelmed with fear, is unable to create an open mind to see that the fear is irrational. Bladder, Kidney's partner, is also being bombarded with the creations of the imagination and is having trouble dealing with impure ideas.

The Liver, receiving no good energy from the Water organs (Kidney and Bladder) is on K-rations of energy and incapable of the foresight to see that the situation will indeed pass. The Heart is trying to coordinate all mental function, which is so out of control that it speeds up—palpitations—trying to sort out the other organs' overload. The Small Intestine, working to discriminate between pure and impure thoughts—or real and unreal—is completely overloaded by the progression of energy coming from Stomach, Large Intestine, Kidney, Bladder, and Liver, as well as being dumped on by the Heart, its partner. Guess what? Diarrhea. The Pericardium, struggling to get a grip on some semblance of rational, sensible sense of self-worth, is on red alert, squeezes the heart, which feels as if the chest is being constricted—which it is—and breathing becomes a problem.

The quickest point to go for during an attack—and the least obvious if you are in public—is Large Intestine 4, Ho Ku. Working it has a general calming effect. Progress through these other points as time and the situation allow: Stomach 36, Kidney 1, Bladder 60, Liver 2, Heart 5 and 7, Small Intestine 4, and Pericardium 9.

For people who are not yet suffering from full-blown biologically-based illness, it may be possible to avert the progression of chemical imbalance in the brain by thinking positive thoughts to counteract the negative one. Suppose depression begins to set in and you know that you have a history of depression. As you begin to sense yourself sinking, force yourself to think a happy thought. "Think about bunny rabbits" as a friend of mine would say, or laugh, because for many years people have known that laughter *is* the "best medicine."

What is more, at the simplest mechanical level, both crying (Lung energy flow) and laughter (Heart energy flow) have been found to increase oxygen to both the brain and the muscles and will temporarily lower high blood pressure. I have successfully used this technique, and so have numerous friends. You only have to try it once to experience the difference in the physical sensations of your body. If you don't like rabbits, think about Sylvester the Cat, Eddie Murphy, Robin Williams, or Whoopi Goldberg—whatever stops the blues or the crazies dead in their tracks and makes you laugh.

In the movie *The Witches of Eastwick*, the three good witches saved themselves from the Devil, when he was trying to kill them, by laughing. Yes, it's just a movie; yet it is a movie with a message, just like the age old classics *Sleeping Beauty*, *Cinderella*, and *The Wizard of Oz*. The message is that love conquers many things. Love, joy, laughter—emotions that have to do with the heart—will heal on many levels.

Laughter—or just pleasant thoughts in the mind—halts the progression of both depression and panic attacks. Some people simply pray for help and the situation is resolved. Once the initial essence of the depression or the panic has been stopped, the problem can then be looked at with a calm rational mind, without sadness or fear.

The associations that you've learned for the Five Elements will also help you symbolically to "see" emotion that is manifesting in a person. View this example in terms of the Five Element animals. A friend suffers from manic depression, and I have noticed over many years that there is a specific pattern creating the depressions.

The first stage involves dwelling on the past. Like an Ox stuck in the mud, memories are clouded by regret, ventures and projects missed out on, and decisions that were made in error circulate through the mind. Regret is associated with the Spleen.

Sadness then enters the arena, like an old Horse put out to pasture. Sadness is the emotion of the Lungs.

Next comes withdrawal in fear and panic that life has been a wasted failure, that business will fall apart and friends will vanish. Like a baby Pig, buried in a mud hollow—in this case, under the blankets in bed—my friend stays hidden away for days,

peeking out at the world only when necessary. Fear is associated with the Kidneys. During this phase of withdrawal, no one
is spoken to, and this can go on for weeks.

Then, all of a sudden, deep grumpiness and anger erupt.
The subconscious goal is the creation of verbal fights—a place
to dump a cesspool of deep-seated anger. This anger has origi-
nated in childhood; the cause for it is either too difficult or too
painful to face. The Liver deals with anger. I will pick up the
telephone and actually *feel* this poor angry, tormented person
on the other end of the line. I know who it is. No matter what
I say, I get ripped to shreds by this Fighting Cock for five or ten
minutes. Having dumped, the telephone is slammed down.

Later, chipper, happy, gentle as a Lamb, my friend is calling
back to ask if I'd like to see a movie or get together for a meal.
Joy and happiness are the emotions of the Heart.

During the cycle of regret-induced depression and assorted other emotions, every negative emotion has moved through
the elements, one by one, and created havoc within the physical body.

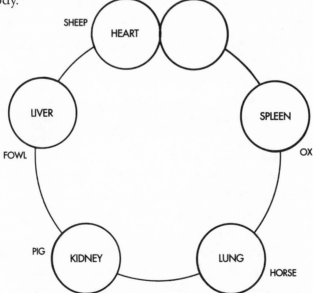

A manic episode moving through the Five Elements

At each emotional stage, this cycle has activated old addictions and compulsive behavior patterns on a physical level: binge and purge eating (Earth), smoking (Metal), and a desire for extra-marital sexual liaisons (Water). After the rage (Wood), and at the end of the negative cycle, there is movement into the positive aspects of emotion (Fire). The acting out is over, and my friend trundles off home to a patient and loving partner.

From manic low to manic high. If this "cycler" were a client, I would work all of the Yin organ points in the ear, and several additional emotional points for balance. This would help to work through the cycle and the deep underlying issues a great deal faster than just "living" through them. For a regimen of specific points to work—both Forbidden Points and non-forbidden—see Part Six, under the heading "Depression."

The time frame for this cycle of regret-induced depression is becoming shorter and shorter due to the real and conscious desire on my friend's part to heal emotional wounds and break old behavior patterns. Although this energetic imbalance is also known as bi-polar depression, or manic-depression, this healing effort is being made without medication, but through the power of the mind, prayer, and a very good psychiatrist—the type who provides tools to work with, rather than creating a dependency on years of office visits.

Several years ago, the withdrawal period would have lasted for weeks or even two months; now it is often down to a day, sometimes only a few hours. The partner has a deep love and a strong will to work through the problems the cycles create; and I feel they will make it as a couple. They both have my deepest respect. The last nine yards are the hardest, and so far, so to speak, the track shoes are still on.

Acupressure and acupuncture can greatly help to eradicate cycles of this nature. Remember, the goal in healing is getting in touch with and releasing the *original* trauma from the body/mind memory. This frees us to truly live and love in the present.

22

addictions and compulsive behavior—why?

IT IS MY BELIEF THAT PHYSICAL ADDICTIONS AND INAPPROPRI-
ate behavioral patterns can be overcome by anyone. Understanding is the key to recovery from addictive behavior. Addictions can have their roots in our inherited genetic makeup or
can stem from our environmental history (such as how we were
treated as children). The origins for addictions are most often
deep within our subconscious.

All addicts—whether addicted to drugs, cigarettes, alcohol,
sex, food, sugar, tea, coffee, gambling, the telephone, shopping,
or another person—are attempting to fill an emotional gap, a
hole, a void within themselves, or are trying to suppress something that is inside of them that is too difficult, too horrible, or
too painful to face.

When the conscious mind understands why we behave the
way we do, then the "will" has a chance to take charge of the
situation and the potential for healing is present. Yet, for the
conscious part of the mind to understand, we first have to access
the subconscious, where the cause of the addiction and resulting self-abuse resides. This cause could be fear, anger/rage, or a
belief system that was programmed into us at an early age.

For example, a programmed belief system could result if a
young boy was aware that his father was unfaithful and had

many affairs, so that at an early age he understands, from his father's example, that monogamy in a relationship is unnecessary. In his adult life he carries on his father's behavioral pattern—acts out—by having numerous sexual liaisons. He is in fact a sex addict and a learned compulsive liar. A loving, stable, committed relationship, which he craves, is always beyond his reach because he continually sabotages the thing he desires most. When he understands the origin of this behavior, he is then equipped to consciously address and change this programmed pattern of being and the way he feels about women in general.

It is now generally accepted that some people will genetically inherit the craving for alcohol; they were born with the blueprint to be alcoholics and are trapped as soon as they take their first curious or social drink as a teenager. Some addictions pass into our bloodstream before birth: some babies are born addicted to cocaine because their mothers are addicted. Others may become alcoholics as a result of childhood trauma, which in turn affects social behavior.

What is it then, to be addicted, to be dysfunctional or codependent? These are three of the most over-used words of the '80s and '90s. What exactly do these three words mean and how do they fit into Traditional Oriental Medicine, founded so long ago?

Addiction

Addiction is simply, or not so simply, a conditioned learned response and way of coping with life. The addiction could be to a person, drug, coffee, tea, sex, gambling, food, shopping, a belief system, a religion, sugar, the telephone, tobacco, or alcohol. Whatever the addiction, addicts feel and believe that they are better equipped to cope with life because of it. It helps them survive. Without it, they go into withdrawal. With it, they live in denial that life is anything but fine. In this state of denial, the addict will often feel trapped and will try to place the blame on someone else rather than look within. Often it takes a serious event, or even hitting rock bottom, to jolt the addict out of denial and get moved toward help.

Dysfunction

When something is dysfunctional, it is not working as it should. The term is also applied to families where life is not quite "right." There is probably abuse—physical, emotional, verbal, religious, sexual—either between parent and parent, parent and child, or child and child. Sometimes, one or both parents turn to their children to fill the gap that the spouse fails to fill. Little girls become surrogate wives, little boys fill daddy's shoes, and both children are shoved into roles they are neither equipped for nor old enough to understand. In a dysfunctional family, the traditional roles are skewed. Children are not cared for and protected as they should be, not allowed to simply be children. Many children take on the role of parent and care for younger brothers or sisters, forced to be responsible "adults" long before it is appropriate. Often these parents abuse alcohol, nicotine, social drugs, or prescription drugs, and were abused themselves as children. Dysfunctional families produce dysfunctional children who often grow into nonfunctioning adults. And unless stopped, it is a cycle that flows from one generation to the next.

Codependency

To be codependent is to rely unreasonably on another person or thing. Codependency comes from programming received in childhood, and results in a person seeking approval—for themselves, for their lives, for often everything they do, say, think, or feel—from someone else.

Codependency involves lack of self-esteem, self-worth,

lack of security from within, and fear. Fear of being alone, fear of not coping, fear of expressing anger or rage (or being unable to do so), fear of losing control of ourselves or someone else, fear of leaving an abusive or painful relationship, fear of having unmet needs yet seeing that everyone else has their needs met, fear of being not good enough, not loveable enough, not rich enough, not famous enough. Codependency keeps us concentrating on the "self," and the result is neurotic self-centeredness, self-serving desires and ways of being. Codependency keeps us focused on the self, the lower self, not the higher spiritual self. Low self-esteem, combined with "not-enough" thoughts, creates individuals who must manipulate and control others so that they can feel superior on some other level, while deep down they feel less-than in everything they do, say, or feel. Enough, enough, enough.

By fully understanding Oriental medicine, we can see how addictions, dysfunction, and codependency come about. They are all based on energy that is grossly out of balance.

Whatever the addictive or dysfunctional pattern, it is physically processed by one of the following organs.

Addiction and Spleen

The Spleen flow regulates the immune system and governs the sex organs in both men and women. To a large extent, addiction to sex results from the desire to love and be loved. There's only one problem: most sex addicts were not loved as children; they may have been starved of love. A small boy may have had a narcissistic, or invasive, or withholding mother. A small girl may have had a cold, withdrawn father. Or perhaps physical, emotional, or sexual abuse played a part in childhood.

The feeling of genuine "love" is unknown. Sex addicts crave love even though they are not too sure what love really is. When we are properly nurtured and loved as children, the result is a peaceful, complete adult who knows that sexual love is an outgrowth of deep spiritual love and commitment, and is a sharing of energies with someone on a Soul level. It is far more than mere orgasm.

From a fear of being alone, sex addicts, like drug addicts, want a quick fix to move them out of boredom, or onto something better, to make them feel happy. The chase, the seduction, and this orgasmic high feeling does not last for long. Uncommitted one-night stands actually help the addict avoid fear of abandonment, fear of engulfment, or fear of true intimacy and commitment. The pull of the sex addiction drive comes from a primal, physical function of a lower nature; there is no higher consciousness involved in this type of sex act.

Some sex addicts will eventually enter into a relationship that has potential for growth and deep intimacy, yet as soon as life becomes too smooth, too happy, too calm—which they perceive as boring—they are off, acting out in pursuit of another sexual conquest.

This can be viewed as Back Flow energy exchange between Spleen and Kidney and the fear associated with Kidney. Why? It depends a great deal on the individual sex addict. This type of behavior often occurs because true intimacy is so frightening that the sex addict pushes away either by withdrawing or being deliberately mean or cruel and causing the partner hurt. The withdrawal may have its roots in family—a parent may have withdrawn—and their present life becomes an endless round of happy-act-out-make-up-happy-act-out *ad infinitum* until the addict becomes seriously involved in a recovery program to get to the bottom of the problem. The codependent partner leaves the relationship and seeks help for their part in the dysfunction and attraction to the addict in the first place. Or the couple stays together and the genuine love that they have on some deep Soul level—damaged Soul recognizing damaged Soul (what really attracted them to each other in the first place)—can help them heal their individual childhood wounds. Doing this consciously as a couple—

focused first on self-love and becoming comfortable with themselves as individuals, leaving blame of the other person out of their thinking, happy with their own company while they each look at, face, and process their own issues—can be very rewarding. While this can result in complete healing, to accomplish it takes enormous patience and dedication to Self and the Other.

The Spleen/Stomach partnership is responsible for the distribution of nourishment, not just physical, food nourishment, but emotional nourishment as well.

So the mouth and stomach are drawn into the drama of the food addict who may binge and purge—bulimia—seeking emotional nourishment through excessive consumption of food with an underlying fear of being fat and the need to control becoming fat. Again, this is a situation of Back Flow energy from Fear and Kidney, or control with Gallbladder. Bulimics often *do* become fat in spite of vomiting their meals because they have disturbed the balance of their digestive enzymes. A great deal of fat is improperly digested in the small intestine.

Anorexics starve themselves because they feel unworthy of love and the nourishment that love—the well-nourished Heart—can bring. Whether it be self-love or love from another person, they fear becoming fat. Even if they achieve skeletal proportions, they still see themselves as fat when they look in the mirror each day, and become obsessed with controlling weight and looks.

Both the bulimic and the anorexic suffer from nutritional imbalance on a broad level. One imbalance leads to another, with potential for manic highs and lows, chemical imbalance in the brain (which can cause depression), food cravings (for proper nourishment), imbalances in the glandular system, and cravings for other substances such as sugar or drugs. It is crucial for those with eating disorders to begin balanced eating habits with nutritional food—breakfast, lunch, afternoon snack, and dinner—and vitamin and mineral supplements taken in doses throughout the day to help restore balance to the physical body so that early aging and degenerative diseases do not take hold.

Addiction and Lungs

Smoking, food binging, telephone-itis, gum chewing, cuticle- and nail-biting, thumb-sucking, nose picking, tobacco chewing, excessive candy chewing and sucking are all oral gratification addictions or compulsive behavior patterns. Smoking satisfies a need stemming from the subconscious desire to numb feelings of grief and sadness, the emotions of the Lung.

The intake of nicotine has a numbing effect on Lung, yet stimulates Heart through the rush of adrenaline released from the adrenal glands, and results in a combined feeling of calm and joy. Other drugs that can be smoked also give this same sense of euphoria because the Heart energy is heightened in an unnatural way. Again the result of the "fix" is Back Flow energy—Lung back to Heart. When people who have smoked marijuana for many years reach what researchers now call "saturation point" (meaning that the body can no longer tolerate marijuana's effects), they often experience severe heart palpitations and sometimes heart attacks. This saturation point differs from individual to individual; what is a long smoking time for one person, is a short time for another.

The Lungs control the Liver, which stores the Blood. If excess energy begins to collect in the Liver because Lung is not functioning properly, this causes old energy to build up and this then affects the Heart, which affects the Liver, which controls the Spleen, and menstrual problems develop with the uterine Blood. The domino effect at work. Just because you started to smoke. Please refer back to the energy exchange charts on pages 59 through 62 in chapter 8 on Five Element Theory. Now are you beginning to see how addictions, energy, and your body all interact?

One of my dearest friends had been smoking for twenty-three years since her college days. She gave up smoking some months ago. Since that time, she has spent countless hours crying, getting in touch with deep sorrow from her childhood. During this period, she has had numerous colds and coughs—the body's way of "crying" and physically releasing sorrow—and, most recently, she suffered from severe bronchitis. One day, after a marathon bout of crying, there were simply no more tears. She said that it felt as if the sun had come out after the desert rains. Then she began to access extreme emotions of anger toward her father. In terms of Five Element Theory, she was unable to fully tap into and begin to release anger toward her father until the last drop of sorrow had left her body. Lung controlling the emotions of Liver.

Once she was able to stay with her anger and direct her rage toward her father, she went through one of the toughest periods in her fourteen years of sobriety. With Liver processing and releasing anger, the urge to drink was tremendous. During this period she had to confront her father with some business problems, and afterward she spent the rest of the day vomiting and was physically and emotionally exhausted. She then took ten days off for a holiday and hid away in seclusion. During this ten-day period she began to look at her tendencies toward anorexia and her improper eating habits—which were all for the purpose of staying thin. She developed the physical symptoms of a stomach ulcer, which proved to be nonexistent. Her intense desire to be in control of her eating, combined with anger and feelings of never being good enough in her father's eyes, led to anorexic behavior. We talked about food, proper portions, and nutritionally balanced meals, and she said that she would really make an effort to eat nutritious meals. Liver/Gallbladder controls Spleen/Stomach.

When she had processed a great deal of anger towards her father (the origins of which she was never quite sure), she began to recall memories of her father abusing her and all her siblings, male and female. With these memories rising from the depths of her unconscious, her life began to swing from powerful-in-control-woman to unsure-hysterical-child plagued by nightmares and panic attacks.

In the relatively short period of nine months, this courageous woman has given up smoking, maintained her sobriety, and come to terms with an eating disorder, "simply" because she was ready to cry for as long as it took to cry and release thirty years of pent up emotions. She laughed and told me, "My body on some level said 'Babe, this is it! No more. I can take no more.'" She is now in the process of selling her house, moving, and changing a career she has had for twenty years. She is finally clear on how she wants to spend the rest of her life and who she wants to let into that life. She is no longer ruled by her father's emotional demands or expectations; she communicates with him as an equal, and finds it "refreshing."

An example of energy medicine at work in the allopathic world of Western medicine is a product called Habitrol. Habitrol is an adhesive nicotine patch, available by prescription, and is reported to stop smoking withdrawal symptoms, enabling the nicotine addict to give up smoking.

Where does the Habitrol patch stick to the body? Right on the upper arm, between points 2 and 3 on the Lung energy flow. Your system is still being bombarded with nicotine, but this time right into the Lung energy flow itself instead of the lung organ. Which is worse? What other flows are in that area of the arm? Large Intestine, Heart, Pericardium, and Small Intestine, not to mention Triple Warmer, which regulates all flows.

The manufacturer's listed side effects from wearing the Habitrol Patch include abdominal pain, constipation, nausea, vomiting, painful menstruation, insomnia, high blood pressure, back pain, nicotine contaminated breast milk, miscarriage, and low birth weight.[1]

1. Basel Pharmaceuticals, division of CIBA-GEIGY Corporation, Summit, NJ. Direct-to-Consumer Advertising, C92-1 (Rev 2/92).

In other words, the placement of the patch directly on the Lung flow is interferring with the natural flow of energy. Who knows how the patch will affect all the other Yin organs—if one considers the Inner Arrow energy flows—or Lung's partner, the Large Intestine? Or the Kidney, to which Lung gives energy? Or the Liver, which Lung controls? Does the Habitrol Patch suppresses Lung to the point that it cannot receive from Spleen? Is that why women have reported menstrual problems? Are these problems due to backed-up energy, which Spleen is unable to pass along to Lung? Only time and Habitrol user observation will tell.

Another example is the Norplant System for birth control. Levonorgestrel implants are surgically placed under the skin in the vicinity of the Heart and Pericardium energy flows. The implants provide five years of protection against pregnancy. Two points along the Pericardium flow are Forbidden Pregnancy Points. Some of the possible side effects from using this implant are high blood pressure, increased risk of blood clotting, heart attack and strokes, irregular menstrual bleeding and delayed disintegration of follicles, increased risk of gallbladder disease, and liver tumors.[2]

Are these side effects and the nearby location of other energy flows a mere coincidence? I believe they are very closely related.

Addiction and Kidney

Any addiction that has a basis of fear will be fueled by Kidney. Kidney is the storehouse for all energy as well as for all sexual energy. Fear is associated with and processed by Kidney.

Kidney is also associated with the will, the ability to make

2. Wyeth-Ayerst Laboratories, Philadelphia. Direct-to-Consumer Advertising © 1993 based on Current Norplant Patient Labeling PI 4069-1, issued December 10, 1990.

decisions and act on these decisions; it is the conductor of energy to our vital soul essence—dwelling within the Liver—and also has to do with the Opening of Passages. If Kidney is blocked with fear, how can we have the will and ambition to change, to open to deeper realms of thought and connect with our Soul or higher consciousness, the part of us that knows we must change old patterns for there to be spiritual growth and right action in our daily lives? When we are blocked by fear, we are trapped in all our addictions and dysfunctional ways. Because Kidney is the storehouse for energy, when Kidney is "off," all flows are in danger of imbalance.

With a reversal of energy pull with Spleen, fear of abandonment can push the sex addict towards casual sex as an outlet for sexual energy. Fear of abandonment or fear of commitment usually pushes the addict to abandon, before he or she can be abandoned. Since Kidney controls Heart, a warm, loving, intimate, and committed relationship can never materialize and the individual continually sabotages, through fears, a real chance at happiness with another individual.

The most troubled person I've counseled was a man who was a classic example of an abused child becoming an addicted adult.

He called me one evening, terrified, suicidal, and wanted to talk. He kept saying, "I think I can talk to you about this, I think I can tell you this; you've been abused, you'd understand . . ." However, when I tried to get him to talk about "this" he refused. When I suggested that he call his family doctor, he became even more frightened. I agreed to see him.

This is an individual who had been abused his whole life, sexually, verbally, and religiously. His mother—a Bible-quoting religious fanatic whose husband had left—made him a surrogate husband at an early age; in fact, they still showered together. Through her indoctrinating religious abuse—where everything is done in the name of "spiritual love"—she had convinced her son that he was the new Christ, and he was, understandably, having a hard time living up to her expectations. He had been sexually abused when he was nine years old by a female baby-sitter. Throughout his school years he had been singled out by female teachers and ridiculed. He usually ended up with girlfriends who treated him terribly.

At this stage of his life he was abusing alcohol, cigarettes, marijuana, cocaine—basically anything that he could get his hands on. His various addictions helped him to "escape" from his life. But these substances also allowed his subconscious memories to surface. On this particular evening, whatever he had taken had freed up these recollections, and they were suddenly making sense to him in a terrifying way.

Facing these memories—facing *fear*—allowed him to release the fear in a healthy, conscious way rather than escape the fear through addictive patterns. That night and into the morning he talked, remembered, cried, and laughed—and it was, for him, the beginning of the healing process.

If someone is consumed by fear and these fears end up putting strain and energetic overload on the Kidney, then the immune system will be affected. Kidney controls Spleen, which governs the immune system. If Kidney is too weak to control, then here again is another domino effect in action.

Fear of losing control will keep the alcoholic glued to his or her bottle of booze, because Kidney, so blocked by fear, cannot give energy to Liver to help end the madness of drinking, to suppress the anger bottled up inside.

Fear of being fat will keep the anorexic starved and the bulimic binging and purging. Fear of failing to keep up appearances of being in control—Gallbladder—will lead to lying and dishonest behavior. Knowing that we have behaved badly will make us feel guilty, judge ourselves, and generally take what we are feeling about ourselves out on someone else, usually the person closest to us at the time—a wife, husband, partner or best friend—or a stranger at the grocery store or in highway traffic.

Fear of losing will keep the gambler gambling, whether it be the horses, dogs, sports events, or high risk investments—the gambler is driven by fear of not having enough, and is anxious for the quick fix, quick money, easy money. Often, through low self-esteem and feelings of worthlessness, the gambler is actually driven by the subconscious desire to *lose,* because he or she feels unworthy of what they have in the first place.

When fear upon fear upon fear have built up, until we are tired, worn out, most likely physically ill, overwhelmed, and can run no more—there stands The Wall, with our issues, our follies, our truths and deceptions written all over it. Then, bottomed out, hopefully we face our addictions one by one, clean up our lives, eat, exercise, and love in an appropriate manner.

The Wall is a painful, fear-filled place to be; it is not about judgment, criticism, or blame of self or others. It just is. It is when you come face to face with an issue that you have silently and secretly in your heart known all along was there. Something from which you will one day no longer be able to run, either physically or emotionally. When we hit The Wall, it is time to become very clear about what we will and will not accept in our lives. Did someone swear at you, punch you, threaten you, lie to you? Does a friend owe you money but will not put that debt down on paper? If you become very clear that these aspects of life are unacceptable to you, they will vanish from your life, these situations will no longer physically manifest in your world.

Pack your bags and run from it, or withdraw from it emotionally and shut down, or ignore it—and it's still there. In front of you—The Wall—to the left—The Wall—to the right—The Wall—turn around—The Wall. On all sides it is there. Once you face your issue, face your fear and accept it, cry through the pain of it—the Lung and Kidney connection—there is a feeling of being alone in the world, yet it is not a scary feeling of "alone." It is peaceful and light, the burden gone. The Wall, once faced, disappears.

Addiction and Liver

As discussed earlier, when we have unreleased anger, it is emotionally assigned to the Liver. A person may develop an alcohol problem due to a subconscious desire to numb the anger, or repress old memories having to do with the original anger.

As the drinker relaxes control (Gallbladder is Liver's partner, and its issue is control), the alcohol allows the anger to come out, and the drinker can become violent while under the influence. "Drowning our sorrows" is a familiar term associated with alcohol oblivion; it shows the relationship between Lung and Liver to help numb feelings. As a Back Flow of energy occurs from Liver to Lung, the Lung pulls in the effect of the alcohol to temporarily obliterate the sadness that Lung is dealing with. Or to quote friend James Wanless in *The Voyager Tarot*, under the card Devil's Play, "When you have too much to drink . . . you become blind and step off your conscious boundaries . . ." [3] The Liver is also associated with the eyes. Many eye problems result from excessive anger, and glaucoma, a condition where pressure builds up in the eye, often leading to blindness, is known as the Devil's Eyes in Oriental medicine.

For someone who fears going to a party or social gathering and who is tongue-tied and inhibited, a drink or two will also disperse the fear in Kidney as the alcohol effect is pulled backwards from Liver.

Some people act out their anger through rape, with the triangular energy exchange between Spleen, governing the sexual organs, Kidney, the storehouse for all sexual energy, and Liver, the processor of anger.

Decision-making, vision (both physical and intuitive), and spirituality are also associated with the Liver. Some people, when under pressure, turn to drinking instead of prayer for guidance and help, and it is generally difficult to be spiritual when angry.

3. James Wanless, *The Voyager Tarot* (Carmel, California: Merrill-West Publishing, 1990)

There is also the rage-aholic; someone who is addicted to rage and full of deep-seated, old (usually childhood) anger. Living with a rage-aholic can be extremely confusing because they have a need to "vent," to get rid of their present anger (which is fueled by a pool of old anger) so they can move into the peace and calm of the Heart. In terms of battering—which is not exclusive to men—this is known as the Cycle of Violence. Rage-aholics generally have a subtle way of baiting the person they are in relationship with (or perhaps working with), a way of asking a subtle question, or making a seemingly harmless statement, such as in the following example:

Rage-aholic: "I just had to pour the grapefruit juice out, it had gone off because you left it out on the counter."

Spouse: "Yeah, I know that's what happens, that's what I keep telling you."

Rage-aholic: "So why did you leave it out?"

Spouse: "I left it out because if I put it in the fridge you complain that it's too cold to drink and you want it left out. So I leave it out even though I know it will go off more quickly than if it was in the fridge."

Rage-aholic: "I only drink the pink grapefruit juice, I don't drink the one you left out. You drink that one, so it should be in the fridge."

Spouse: "I didn't know you only drank the pink one. If you don't drink the other one, how did you know it had gone off?"

Rage-aholic: "That's it, I'm sick of you. You always have to have the last word. Why can't you just shut up? You never know when to stop, do you? I'm not sleeping in here, I can't stand to be near you!" (Leaping out of bed, glaring, while grabbing a pillow, exits the room.)

Spouse: "But . . . but . . . what are you talking about? What on earth is wrong? We were just talking about grapefruit juice!'

Rage-aholic: "Oh shut up, just shut up, you always have to have the last word, don't you. You're always in my face. I can't stand to be near you."

The next day, feeling confused and verbally battered, the spouse will discover that the rage-aholic had an argument earlier that previous afternoon with a business associate, with whom it was impossible to explode. This is typical of many scenes in which a seemingly simple conversation goes from rational discussion to yelling on the rage-aholic's part, which the spouse gets sucked into, out of sheer frustration at trying to understand what on earth is so upsetting. It always ends up with the rage-aholic stomping off into another room, or out of the house altogether, blaming the spouse for the state they are in. Eventually the spouse can recognize the beginning of a mood swing, and choose not to become involved in the insane conversations or take the bait, and the rage-aholic will be left to deal with the anger, alone. You can never win an argument with a rage-aholic, winning is not on their agenda. Dumping blame and yelling is, so save your breath for someone who has more to give or share and less to vent.

Addiction and Heart

Hard core drug addicts who mainline go straight to the source of their pain, via the bloodstream—to their Heart—in an attempt to find joy. Cocaine is also absorbed into the bloodstream via the mucous membrane of the nose when snorted. The nose is part of the respiratory system—Lung—and energy Back Flow from Lung to Heart results in the desired happy "high" effect.

The Heart is responsible for giving energy to Spleen, which governs the sexual organs and the immune system. A Heart that is shut down and unable to feel will also have an effect on general well-being, because it can pull energy from Kidney, the body's storehouse for energy. Our ability to stay well, or become well if we are ill, will be impaired. If the "high" is unable to be maintained, depression can also set in and other addictions will domino into play.

What To Do?

All drugs are either smoked, injected, drunk, snorted, or eaten, and the organs involved in dealing with these drugs are primarily Yin, or female. The Spleen/Pancreas, Lung, Kidney, Liver and Heart are all Yin organs of female energy and emotions. These are all vital organs without which we cannot live. It is our feminine power that gives life in the first place and maintains all of us, whether female or male.

From these Yin organs, men and women derive the ability to nurture, to care, to love, to sustain the life within us through self-love. The gentle, nurturing, compassionate "feeling" side of all men is their Yin side. The ability to embrace the feminine is what maintains a balanced individual.

If, in all honesty, we look at the areas of our lives where we have problems—relationships, food and eating, material possessions, balancing our checkbooks, harming our bodies through cigarette, drug or alcohol abuse, self-destructive behavior—we will begin to identify patterns of behavior that, in a state of total honesty, we cannot ignore. Healing begins when we decide to learn all about ourselves—the deepest, darkest parts—and desire to grow from and with that new knowledge.

Are you an alcoholic because your father was? In simple understanding there comes great healing. It is almost as if the brain takes over and says "OK, I get it, I understand why I send the message to take that drink. Now that I know, I can work with my illness."

When we stop judging ourselves so harshly, we begin to realize that our adult problem areas had their beginnings somewhere in childhood or in our genetic coding; there are no failures in heaven, only in our relatives' houses.

The next time you begin to do something that you know is compulsive, something you do over and over again, simply find a way to stop. Even watching television, videos, and reading books help to suppress emotions or fill a gap. Did you have a nightmare and now the light is on and you're reading? Put the book down and look at the dream. It was only a dream; get out your journal and write about it. Whatever your age, if you have to go back to sleep snuggling your teddy bear then do it, but don't occupy your mind with a book, or pray until the terror of the dream memory goes away. The first time you resist your compulsive behavior is the hardest.

It's like this:

If you are a compulsive shopper—when you start to feel lonely, bored, sad, or nervous, or you think a new outfit, which you neither can afford nor need, will make someone like you more if your relationship is falling apart—then take yourself off to your favorite stores or the mall, knowing that you feel the need to buy. What you are really seeking is self-nurturing, and shopping fills the gap. When you become bored you are really a lost child without direction; shopping brings you back to some sense of center with a focal point. Salespeople sense loneliness, and are more than happy to chat to achieve the sale they want to ring up. I can't remember how many times I've been shopping, and while scrutinizing myself in the mirror, realized that I'd tried on a dress of totally inappropriate color or style and heard a saleslady coo "Daaarling, you look faaabulous!" Too many times for my liking. Fortunately, I have a well-developed sense of what suits me. The point is, no matter how full your closet becomes, you still have an empty space inside your being.

Here is a little exercise that worked for me and a friend who was more of a "problem shopper" than I was. Wander around the stores, look at things and appreciate their beauty without buying anything. Try on scores of dresses and other clothes if you want, but refrain from buying any of them. The first time you do this little exercise it will be hard, yet inside you will feel different. The action of refraining to buy has opened up another circuit in your brain and put you on the road to managing your money in a better way without wasting it. It's as if you've skipped a worn-out groove on a record and hopped into a segment of your brain that's never been used. Pretty soon, you'll be able to wander around, shopping with a friend without buying a single item, help her carry all her shopping bags home, and feel pretty good about yourself in the process.

Now take a look at your childhood from a new perspective. Did someone buy you something every time you started to cry when you were out with your parents? Was there a new toy to shut you up? To calm you down when you began to get angry or agitated on an outing that was going on too long for you as a small child, on "child time"—which seems endless because you are not in control—and did not understand the concept of time in the first place?

Did Daddy spoil you with presents because he felt guilty after he'd molested, beaten, ignored, or yelled at you? Did he buy you expensive gifts for your birthday or for no reason at all? And now, as an adult woman, do you automatically expect your lover or husband to do the same and are always disappointed if they don't; and if they do, you're never satisfied because the gift wasn't big enough, wasn't expensive enough?

It's the same with food or drugs. When you started to whine, did someone buy you an ice cream cone, pop a candy or lollipop into your mouth, and turn you into a sugar freak by the time you were six years old? What sad memory did that deep inhalation of nicotine just stuff back into your body?

Or did you have a childhood where you never had enough and had to do without a great deal of the time? Do you now want to possess everything you see that you like and again you are unsure where the compulsion originates? Do you go to the store to buy one pair of shoes and come home with seven, each in a different color? Look to your early years.

I had a friend who started his childhood off in England. In Britain, going to the pub—a bar that also serves food—is a big thing. Men go for lunch and after work, and families hang out in pubs on the weekends to drink beer or ale, and often to play darts. Pub-crawling is a national pastime. When, as a baby, my friend was taken to the pub with his parents, he was regularly given a sip or two of beer by his dad, especially if he became boisterous or bored with his surroundings. Often, he would turn into the family clown and entertain people with his alcohol-induced antics. As an adult, where does he go to have fun and be joyous? The bar. Does he feel he can be funny without liquor? No, he is tongue-tied and shy. As a baby he was programmed for dysfunctional energetic interplay between Liver, Heart, and Kidney.

By the time he was fourteen, he was a full-blown alcoholic, but he didn't really understand why.

His parents divorced and it was not until he was twenty-one that his mother casually related his early pub history to him. The consequences of that simple confession resulted in a deep anger for what his father had done to him. He instantly hated all women because his mother had not protected him, and from that point on, rarely spoke to his father. For a while he was sailing/drinking his way around the world with his wife, also an alcoholic. They regularly beat each other up. His wife was sexually abused as a child, given alcohol to dope her up, making her drowsy while the abuse took place. Now she gets drunk and wakes up in someone else's bed, not really understanding the whole connection. And her husband is hurt and wonders why his wife is unfaithful. At last report they were back in England seeking professional help with their mutual problem and on the road to Un-covery. Who needs to re-cover anything from childhood? "Recovery" is a grossly misleading word for the subconscious and the brain. They are now a much mellower, more loving couple. For the first time in both their lives they understand why they did the things they did. With that understanding has come the conviction to stop their old ways of relating to each other and the world in general.

Your past is the key to unlocking your present.

23
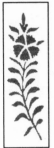
cervical cancer and STDs

ORGANISMS THAT CAN INVADE AND CAUSE ENORMOUS HAVOC within the body are those that attack the sexual organs and create dysfunction. A word of caution. Men can carry sexually transmitted diseases (STDs) such as *Candida albicans* (yeast infections), *Chlamydia trachomatis* (in America alone, over four million people are infected with chlamydia each year), herpes genitalia (HSV II), human papilloma virus (HPV or human wart virus), with *no* symptoms whatsoever.

Gonorrhea and Syphilis

In some cases, gonorrhea and syphilis are also symptomless, and both are among the most damaging of all the sexually transmitted diseases. When symptoms of syphilis are present, they appear within one to twelve weeks after infection and consist of painless sores, usually small. When syphilis goes untreated, the sores turn into a rash, flu-like symptoms appear, with fever, headaches, sore throat. Scarring and blockage of the fallopian tubes (or sperm ducts in men) can occur, which can cause infertility, blindness in your baby at birth, or mental retardation in a developing fetus. In the later stages of syphilis, heart disease, paralysis, and blindness occur. Syphilis, in its later stages, can also cause destruction of the central nervous system and lead to insanity and death. In gonorrhea, an unpleasant vaginal discharge is usually present, and there is pain during intercourse and urination.

Genital warts

Genital warts (condylomata) are small soft growths. According to T. J. Barnett in the *American Medical Association Journal,* "Genital Warts—A Venereal Disease" (Volume 154, 1954, pages 333-34), men who visited the Far East, and had sexual contact, have been known to infect their partners back home with genital warts, yet in some cases the warts took anywhere from three to four weeks to eight months to appear. Sometimes genital warts will grow inward, instead of outward, and cause abscesses in the genital or anal area. Surgery often only permits them to regress further inward and crop up again later on. Vaginal warts can also lead to cervical cancer.

Chlamydia

Chlamydia (pronounced clah-mid-ee-ah) is a bacteria that infects the genitals and occasionally the anus (from anal sex), eyes, and throat (from oral sex). When symptoms are present they include a vaginal discharge that is similar to cottage cheese in appearance and pustulent, pain during menstruation, intercourse, and pain or stinging during urination. Chlamydia can lead to pelvic inflammatory disease (PID), which is extremely serious and involves inflammation of the uterus and the fallopian tubes. PID can lead to sterility or ectopic pregnancies. An ectopic pregnancy occurs in the fallopian tube after fertilization of the egg by the sperm. Instead of traveling down the fallopian tube into the uterus and implanting there, the way it normally would, the fertilized egg implants in the fallopian tube. Ectopic pregnancies are extremely painful and can result in death for mother and/or fetus (baby).

Cervical Cancer

According to Bob Flaws in *Cervical Dysplasia & Prostate Cancer*, the previously mentioned sexually transmitted diseases and virus types have all been linked to cervical cancer, cancer of the prostate, cancers of the skin, tongue, esophagus, anogenital region, and nasopharangeal cavity. Their presence suggests transmission by oral, anal, and genital sex.

The Epstein-Barr virus (EBV) has also been linked to cervical cancer. Each year, nearly half a million women worldwide will develop cervical cancer. Nearly 50 percent of all women who have cervical cancer die within two-and-one-half years of diagnosis.[1] Twenty-five percent of all cervical cancer cases are in women under thirty-five years of age.

There appears to be a link between cervical dysplasia, cervical cancer—a progression of dysplasia—and HPV (human Papilloma virus). I know of a woman who was diagnosed with cervical dysplasia, HPV, and herpes when she was nineteen and still a virgin, having had no known sexual contact with a man. When she was thirty-five, she began to remember being incested by her father who had both HPV and herpes. All of her sisters suffer from cervical dysplasia among other gynecological problems. An entire family was sexually abused by a father. Some of the children have memory of the abuse, however, most are in denial. All have been affected.

There appears to be a mind/body link with this disease, because as this woman moved into therapy and came to terms with her incest issues, her dysplasia disappeared. In terms of Oriental medicine, cervical dysplasia is linked to problems with imbalance of Liver; energy is unable to flow, backs up, become "hot," and stays stuck. I personally would class it as an "angry" disease. In the above case, the woman was an extremely angry

---

1. Bob Flaws, *Cervical Dysplasia & Prostate Cancer* (Boulder, CO: Blue Poppy Press, 1990).

person all around. Known for inappropriate outbursts of rage, she had monumental anger toward her father—can anyone blame her!—all of which began to dissipate during therapy.

She also stopped smoking. As more and more connections are discovered between smoking and disease, one link that has generally become known is the link between smoking and cervical dysplasia and cervical cancer. The Liver, which controls the Spleen (energizer of the sexual organs), is of course controlled by the Lungs. So we have a Controlling Cycle disease here: Lungs to Liver to Spleen.

Through confronting my own incest issues and gynecological problems, and regularly working the Forbidden Pregnancy Points System, I also cleared up a Class III pap smear in under four months.

I would recommend you read Bob Flaws' book if you suffer from this disease. It is well-written, simply explained, and contains a wealth of information, both Western and Eastern.

Hepatitis B

The hepatitis B virus is also spread through sexual contact, and, at present, is the only STD for which a vaccine has been developed. This vaccine is given to sexual partners of those infected with the virus, and is now given to all infants at birth. Hepatitis B is also symptomless in many people who carry the virus. This virus attacks the liver. It can lead to liver failure, liver cancer, brain inflammation, coma, and death. Symptoms occur in three stages, from one to six months after infection. They include flu-like symptoms, vomiting, abdominal pain, diarrhea, nausea, aching joints, chills and/or fever, fatigue and excessive sleepiness, hives, dark urine, light-colored stools, loss of appetite, and a yellowing of the skin and eyes (jaundice). The jaundice stage can last from two to eight weeks. Weight loss is common. The only treatment for hepatitis B is bed rest and healthy nutritious food. Recovery time is about three months.

Herpes

The herpes virus produces sores that are very painful and found in the mouth (as cold sores or fever blisters) and genital region (blisterlike eruptions and ulcerated patches). Herpes is transmitted through active sores in the mouth, vagina, vaginal area, or the penis. There are two types of herpes, Type I (oral) and Type II (genital). Type I used to be linked to fever blisters and cold sores, although it has been found in the genital area as well, spread through oral sex. The symptoms usually appear four to five days after infection. Herpes can be spread to an unborn baby through the birth canal, and can cause infant death. There is no known cure for the herpes virus.

AIDS

Be safe, use condoms. The risk of catching any sexually transmitted disease, let alone AIDS (Acquired Immune Deficiency Syndrome) is just not worth it. It is ill-advised to have sex when you have your period, even if you feel more erotic and sexual at this time; intercourse will reverse the energy flow of the Blood and send it back up and into the womb, causing Stagnation, or old Blood.

The HIV virus, which leads to AIDS, is found in all bodily fluids, including blood, menstrual blood, semen, cervical and vaginal fluids, amniotic fluid, breast milk, mucous discharge, spittal, urine and feces, tears, and perspiration. HIV is spread through unprotected sex (anal or vaginal), needle sharing by drug users, sharing sex toys, and from an infected mother to her unborn child. Tattooing, skin piercing, acupuncture, and electrolysis are all risky if the practitioner does not adequately sterilize his or her equipment.

If you know you have tested positive for HIV or AIDS, you can begin to do something about it by changing your diet and lifestyle—reduce stress, don't overwork, have fun, exercise, get plenty of sleep, stop drinking, smoking, and doing drugs, and do not get any live vaccines. Above all, boost your immune system and your Spleen energy flow. It's a good idea to routinely get a blood test for HIV every six months. After all, you may be in a monogamous relationship *now*, but how many previous lovers have you had? How many sexual partners did your previous lover have *before* you? How many sexual partners has your partner had? And what about the partners' partners? The list of sexual contacts from just one lover could be vast. The disease has been known to take over six years to become active.

Looking at the AIDS problem from a Five Element perspective is helpful. The bodily fluids involved can all be categorized as being associated with Yin organs:

Spleen: blood, menstrual blood, semen, orgasmic discharge in women, amniotic fluid.

Pancreas: Saliva.

Lungs: Mucus

Kidneys: Urine and spittal.

Liver: Tears

Heart: Perspiration

It would appear wise, since the spleen is physically responsible for our immune system, to keep Spleen, above all, healthy, balanced, and capable of passing energy onto the other Yin organs in succession.

Of the Forbidden Pregnancy Points, Stomach 36 can be worked to help boost your immune system. Other points, not forbidden, are listed in the Diagnostic Reference in Part Six. Remember, when you are sexual with someone, you accept their energy into your body; it is more than just physical contact. So, before you make the decision to have sex with someone, get to know them first. Energy is powerful medicine, good and bad.

In chapter 33, "Diet and Fasting," I will discuss how vitamins and the food you eat can help keep your body healthy, and how yeast infections can be eliminated through diet.

24
potency
points
for men

ALTHOUGH THIS MANUAL IS PRIMARILY FOR WOMEN, MANY OF
the women who read and consult it will be in relationships with
men. To optimize the general health, performance, and well-
being of your partner, you might wish to share some parts of
this book with him. For that reason, I am including information
pertinent to men.

Women have come to me doubting their own femininity,
sexual appeal, and wondering "What's wrong with me? Why
isn't he interested in sex anymore? What have I done? Why did
his erection vanish? We used to make love all the time . . . He
gets these night sweats, is it something contagious? Sometimes
I know he has trouble urinating . . ." The problem usually has
nothing to do with the woman, and the man is often just as
confused, even fearful of what is going on within his own body,
embarrassed to even bring up the subject. Sometimes out of
fear, and as a defense mechanism, a man will become moody,
angry, or withdrawn from his partner. While the communication gap widens, he knows there's something wrong. Women
don't hold the monopoly on being confused by their bodily
functions, and a nonperforming penis is harder to ignore, hide,
or to live with than a faked orgasm.

The sexual organ that can be most problematic in the male

is the prostate gland. The prostate, which sits inside the body, just in front of the rectum, below the bladder and surrounding the urethra, can be felt or massaged through the anal opening. The prostate manufactures the alkaline fluid within which the sperm live. If the prostate does not produce enough fluid, the sperm are in a dry river bed. Fertility problems—no sperm, no baby. The most common problems are prostate inflammation and infection, enlargement, cancer and impotence, the inability to maintain an erect penis for intercourse.

In Traditional Oriental Medicine, the prostate is called the "Chamber of Essence." When it becomes inflamed, it causes overall body chills, fever, low back pain, joint and muscle pain, and frequent and urgent need to urinate. If a urinary tract infection is present, there may be pain in the testicles as well. Cancer of the prostate is a slow-growing type of cancer, usually going undetected for a long period. Prostate enlargement will lead to urinary problems, possible burning, difficulty in passing urine, scanty urine flow, and eventual kidney failure. Bowel movements can cause a discharge from the penis. Prostate cancer can hit from the age of 40 onwards, although over 60 is the most common age range. A rectal examination, blood test, and transrectal ultrasound will determine if cancer is present. According to the American Cancer Society, each year 35,000 men die from prostate cancer, and 165,000 more will develop it.

For men with prostate problems, it is important to eat correctly, follow the diet in chapter 33, exercise every day (sitting will aggravate a prostate condition), relax, and refrain from smoking, taking drugs or alcohol, eating spicy or fatty foods.

The typical Yang Excess type of man with a large pot belly is a prime candidate for prostate problems. Slimmer men, who are apt to follow a proper diet and physical fitness program, are often free from prostate illness well into old age (although this is not always true).

Flaxseed oil, fish oils, evening primrose oil, vitamins C and E, selenium, magnesium, zinc, germanium, and the amino acids glycine, alanine, and glutamine (which nourish and energize male cells) have been found to be particularly beneficial to the prostate. Garlic is, of course, excellent since it inhibits infection and has a good supply of vitamins and minerals. Ginseng, ginkgo, saw palmetto, echinacea, pokeweed, mistletoe, and horsetail have also been found to be beneficial for prostate ailments.

Alanine, glycine, and glutamine can be found naturally in a number of foods. *Vegetables*: asparagus, cauliflower, collards, green beans, pumpkin, corn, Chinese cabbage, kale, avocado, potatoes (baked with skins), Romaine lettuce, okra; with lentil sprouts and lima beans having the highest content of all. *Fruits:* dried figs (no additives or preservatives), peaches, pears, and mangoes. *Nuts and seeds:* almonds, sunflower, pumpkin, sesame, and tahini have the highest content.

These amino acids are also found in beef (chuck roast the highest), chicken (breasts and leg), turkey (light meat), fish (notably tuna and clams), pork (ribs, leg, and shoulder), domesticated duck and goose, and wild game (pheasant and quail).

The acupressure points that can be massaged at any time to relieve problems and increase healthy energy within the male body are to be found in Part Five.

Diagnostic
Reference
for
Ailments A-Z

25

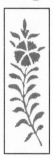

ancient point use rules

IN THE CHAPTER ON FIVE ELEMENT THOUGHT YOU WERE introduced to the concept of the energy flows behaving in a similar way to a river. They have a beginning and an end. At the beginning of the flow the energy is weaker than at the end. There are points along the flows where one flow connects with another, and because they connect they can be used to treat one another.

Like a river, the flows can be regulated in certain places or they can have areas where the energy pools or collects and the energy is very strong. There are places on the river where the flow can be increased if there is too little energy or decreased if there is too much, or where the river meets a large sea, in the case of our body, it is where energy actually meets blood. And there are areas of one river which will effect another river by helping energy to flow in or out of the other.

In this chapter we will look at these Traditional points in their groupings of Source Points, Connecting Points, Accumulation Points, Tonification Points, Sedation or Dispersing Points, Control Points, Controller's Representative Points and Horary Points.

These groupings are actually points and part of traditional theory which are quite complicated, however they are included so that you will be able to see another layer, or depth to the flows for treatment purposes. The reason for this is so that you will have additional points for use to self-correct and balance your flows if you so desire. Points listed in bold are Forbidden Pregnancy Points, and should not be worked if you are pregnant.

Source Points

Source Points along a flow can be thought of as mini "holding tanks," a place where the energy in that flow is held up. The points may be used as diagnosis points; upon touch, they will either feel to have a sufficient or deficient pulse.

FLOW	POINT
Spleen	3
Stomach	42
Lung	9
Large Intestine	**4**
Kidney	3
Bladder	64
Liver	3
Gallbladder	40
Heart	7
Small Intestine	4
Pericardium	7
Triple Warmer	**4**

Connecting Points

The Connecting Points do exactly as their name implies, they connect Yin and Yang organ pairs. They are also known as Luo points. Connecting points can be massaged to help the *partner* in the organ pair. For example, if you had problems and symptoms of imbalance you would massage the Connecting Point of the organ flow which is *worse off,* and this will also help the other organ in the pair.

So, if Spleen was badly imbalanced you would massage Spleen 4 and this would benefit Stomach energy too. Stomach 40 can be massaged to help edema and irregular menstruation; both problems which are associated with Spleen flow imbalance.

FLOW	POINT
Spleen	4
Stomach	40
Lung	**7**
Large Intestine	6
Kidney	**4**
Bladder	58
Liver	5
Gallbladder	37
Heart	5
Small Intestine	**7**
Pericardium	**6**
Triple Warmer	5
Conception Vessel	15
Governing Vessel	1

Accumulation Points

The Accumulation Points are points where energy and blood meet and can be felt to determine if that flow is Excessive or Deficient in energy. They are massaged for treating severe illness. The points which are in brackets are also meeting places on four of the numerous Miscellaneous Channels and are useful for treatments.

FLOW	POINT	
Spleen	8	
Stomach	34	
Lung	6	
Large Intestine	7	
Kidney	5	(K 8, K 9)
Bladder	63	(BL 59)
Liver	6	
Gallbladder	36	(GB 35)
Heart	6	
Small Intestine	6	
Pericardium	4	

Tonification Points

A Tonification Point is a point on an energy flow, which when massaged will increase, or draw energy into that flow. The point should be massaged in a clockwise direction.

Along each flow there is a point which I like to define as an Ancestor Point. Remember the Parent and Child rule? Well, in Classical terms, it is said that each organ flow has an Element Point along that flow.

So you would have an Earth, Fire, Wood, Water and Metal point for example, on Spleen flow. The Earth Point on Earth element Spleen would be the Child or Self Point and it is also known as the Horary Point. By definition, an Horary Point is a point on a flow which is said to be most powerful during the peak hours of that flow; in Spleen's case it would be 9-11 a.m. The *Horary Point of the Parent Organ Flow* should also be massaged when working a Tonification Point. Why? Because a Parent Organ gives to a Child Organ.

FLOW	POINT	PARENT/HORARY POINT	
Spleen	2	Heart	8
Stomach	41	Small Intestine	5
Lung	9	Spleen	3
Large Intestine	4	**Stomach**	**36**
Kidney	7	Lung	8
Bladder	67	Large Intestine	1
Liver	8	Kidney	10
Gallbladder	43	Bladder	66
Heart	9	Liver	1
Small Intestine	3	Gallbladder	41
Pericardium	9	Liver	1
Triple Warmer	3	Gallbladder	41

Sedation Points

Sedation or Dispersing Points are points which when massaged in a counter clockwise direction will disperse energy from that particular flow. They are powerful clear-out points. It is also helpful to massage the Horary Point of the Child Organ Flow. Why? Because a Child Organ takes energy from the parent.

FLOW	POINT	CHILD/HORARY POINT	
Spleen	5	Lung	8
Stomach	**45**	Large Intestine	1
Lung	5	Kidney	10
Large Intestine	**2**	Bladder	66
Kidney	1	Liver	1
Bladder	65	Gallbladder	41
Liver	2	Heart	8
Gallbladder	38	Small Intestine	5

FLOW	POINT	CHILD/HORARY POINT	
Heart	7	Spleen	3
Small Intestine	8	**Stomach**	**36**
Pericardium	7	Spleen	3
Triple Warmer	10	**Stomach**	**36**

Dispersing the Earth (child) point of the Fire (parent) Meridian—Heart 7—will disperse both Heart and Spleen. Massaging the Earth (parent)—Lung 9—and Water (child)—Lung 5—points of the Metal flow or the Fire (parent)—Spleen 2—and Metal (child)—Spleen 5—points of the Earth flow will stimulate and regulate the flow itself (Earth) as well as the parent (Fire) and child (Metal) flows.

It's a bit like the children's ball game "Pig in the Middle." The Element in the middle will be affected by and affect the Elements on either side of it. If the "Pig" has the ball (energy), he's taken it from the other two. If one person has the ball, the other two do not.

However, there is an important treatment method to take into account. The rule relating to Sedation, or Dispersion of old energy is this:

- Excess Earth equals Deficient Water, therefore Tonify Wood.
- Excess Metal equals Deficient Wood, therefore Tonify Fire.
- Excess Water equals Deficient Fire, therefore Tonify Earth.
- Excess Wood equals Deficient Earth, therefore Tonify Metal.
- Excess Fire equals Deficient Metal, therefore Tonify Water.

This is an exchange between Child (excess) and Great Grandparent (deficient) and Grandparent (tonify). In bringing energy into the Grandparent element, the Child and Great Grandparent are balanced. A generational go-between.

Control Points

The Control point or Grandparent Point within a flow will control or regulate the energy along that flow.

FLOW	POINT	ELEMENT
Spleen	1	Wood point
Stomach	43	Wood point
Lung	10	Fire point
Large Intestine	5	Fire point
Kidney	3	Earth point
Bladder	40	Earth point
Liver	4	Metal point
Gallbladder	44	Metal point
Heart	3	Water point
Small Intestine	2	Water point
Pericardium	3	Water point
Triple Warmer	2	Water point

Controller's Representative

The Controller's Representative or Grandparent Point outside an element is used in conjunction with the Control Point within an element. Both Points—Control and Controller's Representative—are used when sedating or tonifying a flow. These Grandparent points outside the flow to be treated are also Horary points in their own right. A Horary Point on the

Grandparent flow can be used to move energy in the Grand-child flow.

FLOW	GRANDPARENT/POINT	
Spleen	Liver	1
Stomach	Gallbladder	41
Lung	Heart	8
Large Intestine	Small Intestine	5
Kidney	Spleen	3
Bladder	**Stomach**	**36**
Liver	Lung	8
Gallbladder	Large Intestine	1
Heart	Kidney	10
Small Intestine	Bladder	66
Triple Warmer	Bladder	66
Pericardium	Kidney	10

26

 *different problems, different points*

THIS CHAPTER BRIEFLY DEALS WITH PROBLEMS YOU MAY BE faced with from time to time. Little ailments, big ailments, physical, emotional; a bit of this and a bit of that. Obviously, this subject alone could fill an entire book just on ailments and traditional treatment points; I have tried to give a well-rounded list, which I hope will help most women on a day-to-day basis.

This list also serves a diagnostic function: If you are attempting to read yourself to determine which flow is blocked in terms of energy, it is helpful to turn to a list of symptoms. If, for example, you are suffering from acne, constipation, and exhaustion, you will find that all share Large Intestine Flow, and this flow should be a clue as to what flows may be next affected, and to other areas that may be a problem.

The Forbidden Pregnancy Points, where they appear from time to time in this list, are printed in bold to remind you not to stimulate them if you are pregnant, and wish to remain so.

Sedation (counterclockwise) and tonification (clockwise) are specified where they are an important aspect of the point work.

Keep in mind that working the points should not replace traditional medical treatment. In all cases, if your problems persist or are very serious, consult your regular doctor.

ACNE, PREMENSTRUAL:
Small Intestine

    4   *Wrist Bone*

Large Intestine

    20   *Welcome Fragrance*

Conception Vessel

    24   *Sauce Receptacle or*
                        Receiving Fluid or Celestial Pool

ADRENAL DEFICIENCY:
Spleen

    6   ***Three Yin Crossing***

Kidney

    7   ***Returning Flow***

Bladder

    52   *Will Chamber or Palace of Essence*

Conception Vessel

    6   *Sea of Ch'i*

Governing Vessel

    4   *Life Gate*

AGORAPHOBIA (*see anxiety*)

ALLERGIES:
Large Intestine

    4   ***Ho Ku*** *or Tiger's Mouth or*
                        Joining the Valleys or
                        Great Eliminator

Large Intestine

    11   *Crooked Pond*

Kidney

    27   *Store House*

Triple Warmer

    5   *Outer Frontier Gate*

ANGER, INTENSE:
Kidney
   3   *Greater Mountain Stream*
Bladder
   65   *Bone Binder*
Liver
   3   *Supreme Rushing or Great Pouring*
                 or Great Surge
   8   *Crooked Spring*
Gallbladder
   40   *Wilderness Mound*
Pericardium
   9   *Rushing into the Middle*
Governing Vessel
   12   *Body Pillar*

ANTIMISCARRIAGE: *See Appendix B*

ANXIETY:
Stomach
   36   **Leg Three Miles**
Large Intestine
   4   **Ho Ku**
Kidney
   1   **Bubbling Spring**
Bladder
   60   *Kunlun Mountains*
Liver
   2   *Moving Between*
Heart
   5   *Connecting Grain*
   7   *Spirit Gate*
Small Intestine
   4   *Wrist Bone*
Pericardium
   9   *Central Hub*

ANTICONVULSIVE:
Conception Vessel
15   *Turtledove Tail or Spirit Mansion*

APATHY:
Stomach
41 *(tonify)*   *Ravine Divide*
Kidney
4   *Great Bell*
Gallbladder
38*(sedate)*   *Yang's Support*

BACKACHE:
Bladder
38   *Superficial Gate*
42   *Spiritual Soul Gate*
47   *Soul Gate*
Gallbladder
30   *Jumping Circle*
Triple Warmer
15   *Heavenly Bone-Hole*
Governing Vessel
2   *Lumbar Shu*
4   *Life Gate*

BEE STING:
Kidney
6   *Shining Sea*
Bladder
64   *Capital Bone*

BONES, BRITTLE:
Kidney
3 *(tonify)*   *Great Ravine*
7   ***Returning Flow***

Bladder

23	*Kidney's Hollow (Shu)*
52	*Will Chamber or Palace of Essence*

Conception Vessel

4	*Origin Pass or Cinnabar Field or Essential Dew*

BREASTS, LUMPS *(and Implant Problems)*
Spleen

4	*Prince's Grandson*

Small Intestine

3	*Back Ravine*

BREASTS, SORE :
Stomach

13	*Ch'i Door*
16	*Breast Window*
18	*Breast Root*

Kidney

22	*Corridor Walk or Walking Gentleman*

BREATH, SHORTNESS OF:
Kidney

3 *(tonify)*	*Great Ravine*

Bladder

15	*Heart's Hollow (Shu)*
23	*Kidney's Hollow (Shu)*

Heart

7 *(tonify)*	*Spirit Gate*

BROKEN HEART:
Heart

1	*Highest Spring*
7	*Spirit Gate*

BROKEN HEART (CONT):
Pericardium

    7   *Great Mound*

CLAUSTROPHOBIA:
Spleen

    6   **Three Yin Crossing**

    10   *Sea of Blood*

Bladder

    17   *Diaphragm Hollow (Shu)*

Heart

    7   *Spirit Gate*

COLDS AND FLU:
Kidney

    27   *Hollow Residence*

Bladder

    3   *Eyebrow's Pouring*

    47   *Soul Gate*

Triple Warmer

    15   *Celestial Bone Hole*

Governing Vessel

    14   *Great Hammer*

CONFUSION:
Large Intestine

    4   **Ho Ku**

    11   *Crooked Pond*

CONSTIPATION:
Stomach

    25   *Heavenly Pivot*

Large Intestine

    4   **Ho Ku**

Conception Vessel

 12   *Middle Duct*

CRAMPS, MENSTRUAL:

Spleen

 3   *Supreme White*

 6   ***Three Yin Crossing or***
          Life Support

 12   *Rushing Gate*

 13   *Bowel Abode*

Stomach

 42   *Rushing Yang*

Bladder

 47   *Soul Gate*

Liver

 2   *Walk Between*

 3   *Supreme Rushing or Great Pouring*
          or Great Surge

 6   *Middle Capital*

Conception Vessel

 4   *First Gate*

DEPRESSION:

Spleen

 6   ***Three Yin Crossing***

Stomach

 41   *Ravine Divide or Released Stream*

Large Intestine

 6   *Side Passage*

 11   *Crooked Pond*

Kidney

 3   *Great Ravine*

 6   *Shining Sea*

Bladder

 67   *Extremity of Yin*

DEPRESSION (CONT):

Liver

2	*Moving Between*
3	*Supreme Rushing or Great Pouring or Great Surge*
8	*Crooked Spring*

Gallbladder

34	**Yang Mound Spring**
38	*Yang Support*
40	*Wilderness Mound*

Heart

3	*Little Sea*
9	*Little Rushing In or Lesser Surge*

Small Intestine

3	*Back Ravine*
4	*Wrist Bone*
7	**Regulating Branch or Branch to the Correct**

Triple Warmer

3	*Middle Islet*

Governing Vessel

13	*Kiln Path or Way of Happiness*

DISHARMONY, PARTNER:

Pericardium

6	**Inner Frontier Gate**

EARACHE:

Large Intestine

4	**Ho Ku**

Small Intestine

3	*Back ravine*

Triple Warmer
>   *4*   *Yang Pond*

EDEMA: *See Appendix B*

ENERGY, BOOST WHILE JOGGING:
Stomach
>   *36*   *Leg Three Miles*

ENERGY, LOW:
Bladder
>   23   *Kidney's Hollow (Shu)*
>   31   *Upper Bone Hole*
>   39   *Crooked Yang*

EXHAUSTION, PHYSICAL AND MENTAL:
Large Intestine
>   15   *Shoulder Bone*
Kidney
>   3   *Great Ravine*
Bladder
>   17   *Diaphragm Hollow (Shu)*
>   39   *Crooked Yang*
>   58   *Taking Flight or Soaring*
Heart
>   3   *Little Sea*
Triple Warmer
>   3   *Middle Islet*

FAINTING:
Stomach
>   *36*   *Leg Three Miles*
Large Intestine
>   *4*   *Ho Ku*
Heart
>   1   *Highest Spring*
>   7   *Spirit Gate*

FEAR OF THE FUTURE:
Kidney

4	***Great Bell***
Bladder	
62	*Extending Vessel*
Heart	
5	*Connecting Grain*
7 (sedate)	*Spirit Gate*
Pericardium	
6	*Inner Frontier Gate*

FERTILITY, INCREASE:
Spleen

3	*Supreme White*
Large Intestine	
11	*Crooked Pond*
Kidney	
3	*Greater Mountain Stream*
Triple Warmer	
7	*Assembly of Ancestors*
Conception Vessel	
3	*Utmost Middle*

FOOD POISONING:
Stomach

30	*Surging Ch'i*
Lung	
9	*Great Abyss*
Large Intestine	
4	***Ho Ku***
Bladder	
59	*Instep Yang*
60	*Kunlun Mountains*

Gallbladder
40   *Hill Ruins*

HANGOVER:
Stomach
45   *Severe Mouth*

HAIR LOSS:
Kidney
3   *Great Ravine*
7   ***Returning Flow***
Bladder
52   *Will Chamber or Palace of Essence*
Conception Vessel
4   *Origin Pass or Cinnabar Field or*
                     Essential Dew

HEADACHES:
Stomach
1   *Receive Tears*
Gallbladder
1   *Orbit Bone or Pupil Bone-Hole*
20   *Wind Pond*
Bladder
1   *Eyes Bright*
2   *Collect Bamboo*

HEART PALPITATIONS:
Bladder
15   *Heart's Hollow (Shu)*
Heart
7   *Spirit Gate*
Conception Vessel
6   *Sea of Ch'i*
14   *Great Tower Gate*

HYSTERIA:
Stomach

	40	*Abundant Bulge*
	42	*Surging Yang*

IMMUNE SYSTEM, STRENGTHEN:
Stomach

	36	**Leg Three Miles**

Large Intestine

	11	*Crooked Pond*

Kidney

	27	*Store House*

(Colds and coughs)
Bladder

	23	*Kidney's Hollow (Shu)*
	36	*Near Division*

(Colds and Flu)
Bladder

	47	*Soul Gate*

Liver

	3	*Supreme Rushing or Great Pouring or Great Surge*

Triple Warmer

	5	*Outer Frontier Gate*

Conception Vessel

	6	*Sea of Ch'i*

Conception Vessel

	17	*Within the Breast (Thymus gland)*

INDIFFERENCE:
Lung

	7	**Broken Sequence**

INDIGESTION:
Stomach

36	*Leg Three Miles*
45	*Severe Mouth*

INFERTILITY:
Bladder

33	*Middle Sacral Bone-Hole*
34	*Lower Sacral Bone-Hole*

Conception Vessel

4	*Origin Pass or Cinnabar Field or Essential Dew*
6	*Sea of Ch'i*
7	*Yin Intersection*

INSOMNIA, DUE TO TENSION:
Spleen

2	*Great Capital*
6	*Three Yin Crossing*

Stomach

8	*Head Support*
40	*Abundant Splendor*

Bladder

10	*Heavenly Pillar*
38	*Superficial Cleft*
62	*Extended Vessel*

Kidney

1	*Bubbling Spring*
4	*Great Bell*
6	*Shining Sea*

Liver

2	*Moving Between*

INSOMNIA (CONT):

Liver

3	*Supreme Rushing or Great Pouring or Great Surge*

Gallbladder

20	*Wind Pond*

Heart

7	*Spirit Gate*

KNEE PAIN:

Spleen

9	**Yin Mound Spring**

MALE PROBLEMS:

(Impotence):

Spleen

12	*Rushing Gate*
13	*Bowel Abode*

Stomach

36	**Leg Three Miles**

Kidney

1	**Bubbling Spring**

Bladder

23	*Kidney's Hollow (Shu)*
29	*Middle Backbone Shu*
30	*White Ring Shu*
47	*Soul Gate*

Liver

8	*Crooked Spring*

Triple Warmer

4	**Yang Pond**

(Prostate Problems)
   Conception Vessel
      1   *Meeting of Yin*
      2   *Crooked Bone*
   Kidney
      11   *Transverse Bone*

(Semen Leakage):
   Kidney
      3   *Greater Mountain*
                        Stream

(Testes)
   Stomach
      30   *Surging Ch'i*
   Conception Vessel
      3   *Central Pole or Jade Spring*
      4   *Origin Pass or Cinnabar*
                        Field or Essential Dew
   Governing Vessel
      14   *Great Hammer*

MELANCHOLY:
   Spleen
      2   **Great Capital**
   Kidney
      1   **Bubbling Spring**
      6   *Shining Sea*
   Gallbladder
      38 (sedate)   *Yang Support*
   Heart
      3   *Little Sea*
      7   *Spirit Gate*

MELANCHOLY (CONT):

Small Intestine

3		*Back Ravine*
4		*Wrist Bone*

Triple Warmer

3		*Middle Islet*

MEMORY

Governing Vessel

4	*Life Gate*
20	*One Hundred Convergences*
24.5	*Third Eye*

Governing Vessel

26	*Water Trough or Middle of Man*

Bladder

10	*Heavenly Pillar*
43	*Yang's Parameter*

Gallbladder

20	*Wind Pond*

MENOPAUSE:

(Hot Flashes)

Stomach

36	*Leg Three Miles*
43	*Sunken Valley*

Large Intestine

4	*Ho Ku*

Bladder

31	*Upper Bone Hole*
66	*Penetrating Valley*

Kidney

1	*Bubbling Spring*
3	*Greater Mountain Stream*

27	*Store House*
Gallbladder	
20	*Wind Pond*
Triple Warmer	
3	*Middle Islet*
Conception Vessel	
17	*Within the Breast*

(Tinnitus)

Triple Warmer	
5	*Outer Frontier Gate*
17	*Wind Screen*
18	*Spasm Vessel*
20	*Small Ear Angle*
21	*Ear Gate*
22	*Harmony Bone-Hole*
Large Intestine	
4	***Ho Ku***
Kidney	
6	*Shining Sea*
Bladder	
47	*Soul Gate*
Gallbladder	
2	***Hearing Assembly***
20	*Wind Pond*
Small Intestine	
4	*Wrist Bone*
19	*Listening Palace*
Pericardium	
6	***Inner Frontier Gate***
8	***Palace of Weariness***

MENOPAUSE (CONT):

(Stop Perspiration)
Kidney

3	*Great Ravine*
7	***Returning Flow***

Bladder

15	*Heart's Hollow (Shu)*
23	*Kidney's Hollow (Shu)*

Heart

7	*Spirit Gate*

(Urinary Incontinence):
Bladder

20	*Spleen's Hollow (Shu)*

Governing Vessel

20	*One Hundred Convergences*

(Uterine Prolapse):
Stomach

36	***Leg Three Miles***

Bladder

20	*Spleen's Hollow (Shu)*

Liver

13	*System's Door*

Conception Vessel

12	*Supreme Granary*

MIGRAINES:
Liver

2	*Moving Between*
14	*Cycle Gate*

Gallbladder

20	*Wind Pond*
34	***Yang Mound Spring***

Also try: Stomach 8, Large Intestine 4, and Gall Bladder 39.

NAUSEA:
    Spleen
        3   *Supreme White*
    Stomach
        42   *Rushing Yang*
    Liver
        3   *Supreme Rushing or*
                       Great Pouring or Great Surge

NIGHTMARES:
    Spleen
        5   *Merchant Mound*

OBSESSIONS:
    Spleen
        5   *Merchant Mound*
    Large Intestine
        4   ***Ho Ku***
    Bladder
        62   *Extending Vessel*
    Pericardium
        7   *Great Mound*

OVARIES:
    Spleen
        6   ***Three Yin Crossing or***
                       Life Support

    Kidney
        2   ***Blazing Valley or***
                       Dragon in the Abyss
        13   *Ch'i Door*
    Governing Vessel
        4   *Life Gate*

OVEREXCITEMENT:
Stomach

42 (sedate)	*Surging Yang*
45 (sedate)	**Severe Mouth**

Bladder

67	*Reaching Yin*

PANCREAS:
Spleen

3	*Supreme White*

Bladder

20	*Spleen's Hollow*

Triple Warmer

3	*Middle Islet*

PERSECUTION COMPLEX:
Gallbladder

34	**Yang Mound Spring**

PREOCCUPIED:
Lung

9	*Great Abyss*

Liver

6	*Middle Capital*

PREGNANCY:

(Morning Sickness):
Conception Vessel

12	*Middle Duct*

Kidney

21	*Dark Gate*

(Stop a Premature Delivery):
Conception Vessel
    3   *Utmost Middle or Central Pole*
Kidney
    9   *Building Guest or Attack Expulsion*

(Turn a Breech Presentation):
Bladder
    67   *Extremity of Yin*

(To Induce Labor)
Bladder
    31   *Upper Bone Hole*
    32   *Second Bone Hole*
Large Intestine
    4   ***Ho Ku***
Spleen
    6   ***Three Ying Crossing or Life Support***

(To Dilate the Cervix):
Triple Warmer
    6   *Branch Ditch*
Conception Vessel
    4   *First Gate*
Liver
    2   *Walk Between*
    3   *Supreme Rushing or Great Pouring or Great Surge*
Spleen
    6   ***Three Yin Crossing***
Gallbladder
    34   ***Yang Mound Spring***
Large Intestine
    4   ***Ho Ku***

(To Dilate the Cervix, cont.):
Stomach
36	*Leg Three Miles*

(Anxiety During Labor):
Heart
5	*Penetrating Inside*
7	*Spirit Gate*

(Calm Fetus and Help Labor):
Bladder
67	*Extremity of Yin*

(Lower Back Labor Pains):
Bladder
32	*Second Sacral Bone-Hole*
33	*Middle Sacral Bone-Hole*
34	*Lower Sacral Bone-Hole*
60	*Kunlun Mountains*

(Birthing, Once Labor Has Started):
Gallbladder
21	*Shoulder Well*

Liver
6	*Middle Capital*

Small Intestine
8	*Small Sea*

Large Intestine
4	*Ho Ku*

Bladder
67	*Extremity of Yin*

(Points after the Birth is Over):
Spleen
3	*Supreme White*

Stomach
    42   *Rushing Yang*

Gallbladder
    40   *Wilderness Mound*

Pericardium
    7   *Great Mound*

Governing Vessel
    2   *Lower Back's Hollow*
    4   *Life Gate*

POSTPARTUM PAIN:

Conception Vessel
    2   *Crooked Bone*
    4   *First Gate*

Stomach
    29   *The Return*
    30   *Ch'i Rushing*

Kidney
    14   *Fourfold Fullness*

Bladder
    31   *Upper Sacral Bone-Hole*
    32   *Second Sacral Bone-Hole*

Governing Vessel
    20   *One Hundred Convergences*

NURSING:

(Milk Producing):
Conception Vessel
    17   *Within the Breast*

Small Intestine
    1   *Little Marsh*
    2   *Forward Valley*

Stomach
    13   *Ch'i Door*

(Milk Producing, cont.):
Stomach

16	*Breast Window*
18	*Breast Root (stops breast abscess)*

Lung

1	*Middle Palace*

Kidney

22	*Corridor Walk or Walking Gentleman*

Gallbladder

20	*Wind Pond*

Liver

3	*Supreme Rushing or Great Pouring or Great Surge*

Small Intestine

1	*Little Marsh (stops breast abscess)*

(Weaning and to Stop Lactation):
Gallbladder

37	*Bright and Clear*
41	*Foot Overlooking Tears*

Small Intestine

1 (sedate)	*Little Marsh*
2 (sedate)	*Forward Valley*

Conception Vessel

3 (sedate)	*Utmost Middle*

Bladder

22 (sedate)	*Triple Burner's Hollow*
51 (sedate)	*Prosperous Gate*

POSTPARTUM DEPRESSION:
Small Intestine

1	*Little Marsh*

SADNESS:
Spleen
3   *Supreme White*
Heart
3   *Little Sea*
9   *Lesser Surge*
Small Intestine
3   *Back Ravine*
Triple Warmer
3   *Middle Islet*
Governing Vessel
13   *Kiln Path or Way of Happiness*

SELF-DOUBT:
Bladder
15   *Heart's Hollow (Shu)*
39   *Crooked Yang*

SEXUAL OBSESSION:
Pericardium
6   ***Inner Frontier Gate***
7   *Heart Governor*
9   *Central Hub*
Conception Vessel
7   *Yin Intersection*

SHOCK:
Lung
9   ***Great Abyss***
Kidney
1   ***Bubbling Spring***
Heart
7   *Spirit Gate*

THYROID, ENLARGED:

Stomach	
9	*Man's Welcome*
Large Intestine	
4	**Ho Ku**
Bladder	
15	*Heart's Hollow (Shu)*
Heart	
7	*Spirit Gate*
Conception Vessel	
22	*Celestial Chimney*

27

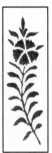 *patterns of illness interchange*

WITHIN THE BODY, ENERGY FLOWS FROM ONE FLOW AND organ to the next, in sequences of imbalance. In recognizing and following the patterns, we can take action to stop further progression of any negative energy influences (illness) within the body, by knowing where imbalance may hit and domino next. The patterns can be "seen" in familiar shapes when laid out in "clock" formation, and they also contain subpatterns, within the main pattern. These flows can go in both a clockwise and counterclockwise direction.

△ *pattern*

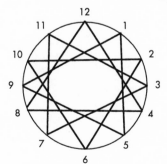

In organ order of normal energy exchange around the circle, the main energetic domino effect in this pattern would be as follows and reads down each column:

LU	LI	ST	SP	HT	SI	BL	K	P	TW	GB	LV
HT	SI	BL	K	P	TW	GB	LV	LU	LI	ST	SP
P	TW	GB	LV	LU	LI	ST	SP	HT	SI	BL	K

The subset follows within each particular organ:

LU	LU	LU	LI	LI	LI
SI	BL	K	BL	K	P
TW	GB	LV	GB	LV	LU

SP	SP	SP	ST	ST	ST
P	TW	GB	K	P	TW
LU	LI	ST	LV	LU	LI

HT	HT	HT	SI	SI	SI
TW	GB	LV	GB	LV	LU
LI	ST	SP	ST	SP	HT

K	K	K	BL	BL	BL
LU	LI	ST	LV	LU	LI
HT	SI	BL	SP	HT	ST

TW	TW	TW	P	P	P
ST	SP	HT	LI	ST	SP
B	K	P	SI	BL	K

LV	LV	LV	GB	GB	GB
HT	SI	BL	SP	HT	SI
P	TW	GB	K	P	TW

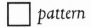 *pattern*

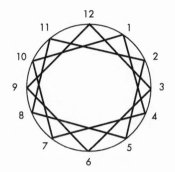
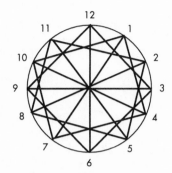

Here is another pattern of energy flow, and like the previous pattern, is read down the column.

LU	LI	ST	SP	HT	SI	BL	K	P	TW	GB	LV
SP	HT	SI	BL	K	P	TW	GB	LV	LU	LI	ST
BL	K	P	TW	GB	LV	LU	LI	ST	SP	HT	SI
TW	GB	LV	LU	LI	ST	SP	HT	SI	BL	K	P

The subset follows:

LU	SP	BL	TW
SP	BL	TW	LU
BL	TW	LU	SP

☯

LI	HT	K	GB
HT	K	GB	LI
K	GB	LI	HT

ST	SI	P	LV
SI	P	LV	ST
P	LV	ST	SI

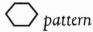 *pattern*

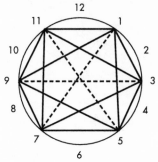

This is a pattern of flow imbalance that has four levels to it. The first level indicates a progressed imbalance in six out of twelve flows and organs and would involve a highly complex set of symptoms.

LU	LI	ST	SP	HT	SI	BL	K	P	TW	GB	LV
ST	SP	HT	SI	BL	K	P	TW	GB	LV	LU	LI
HT	SI	BL	K	P	TW	GB	LV	LU	LI	ST	SP
BL	K	P	TW	GB	LV	LU	LI	ST	SP	HT	SI
P	TW	GB	LV	LU	LI	ST	SP	HT	SI	BL	K
GB	LV	LU	LI	ST	SP	HT	SI	BL	K	P	TW

The second level subset follows:

LU	LI	ST	SP	HT	SI	BL	K	P	TW	GB	LV
HT	SI	BL	K	P	TW	GB	LV	LU	LI	ST	SP
P	TW	GB	LV	LU	LI	ST	SP	HT	SI	BL	K

The third level subset follows:

LU	LU	LU	LU	LU	LU
HT	ST	ST	P	GB	GB
BL	BL	P	BL	BL	HT

☯

ST	ST	ST	ST	ST	ST
BL	HT	HT	GB	LU	LU
P	P	GB	P	P	BL

☯

HT	HT	HT	HT	HT	HT
P	BL	BL	LU	ST	ST
GB	GB	LU	GB	GB	P

☯

BL	BL	BL	BL	BL	BL
GB	P	HT	HT	ST	P
LU	LU	GB	LU	LU	ST

☯

P	P	P	P	P	P
HT	BL	GB	LU	GB	BL
ST	ST	HT	ST	ST	LU

☯

GB	GB	GB	GB	GB	GB
ST	LU	P	BL	P	LU
HT	BL	ST	HT	HT	HT

The fourth level subset follows:

LU	ST	LU
HT	HT	ST
BL	P	BL
GB	GB	P

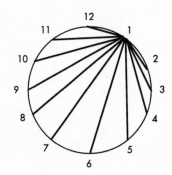

⌐ *pattern*

This is a pattern with two levels, the main and the subset:

LU	LI	ST	SP	HT	SI	BL	K	P	TW	GB	LV
BL	K	P	TW	GB	LV	LU	LI	ST	SP	HT	SI
LI	ST	SP	HT	SI	BL	K	P	TW	GB	LV	LU

The subset follows:

LU	LU	LU	LU	LU	LU	LI	LI	LI	LI	LI	LI
LV	GB	TW	P	K	BL	ST	SP	HT	SI	BL	K
BL	SI	HT	SP	ST	LI	P	TW	GB	LV	LU	ST

SP	SP	SP	SP	SP	SP	ST	ST	ST	ST	ST	ST
TW	GB	LV	LU	LI	ST	P	TW	GB	LV	LU	LI
HT	SI	BL	K	P	TW	SP	HT	SI	BL	K	P

☯

HT	HT	HT	HT	HT	HT	SI	SI	SI	SI	SI	SI
GB	LV	LU	LI	ST	SP	LV	LU	LI	ST	SP	HT
SI	BL	K	P	TW	GB	BL	K	P	TW	GB	LV

☯

K	K	K	K	K	K	BL	BL	BL	BL	BL	BL
LI	ST	SP	HT	SI	BL	LU	LI	ST	SP	HT	SI
P	TW	GB	LV	LU	LI	K	P	TW	GB	LV	LU

☯

TW	TW	TW	TW	TW	TW	P	P	P	P	P	P
SP	HT	SI	BL	K	P	ST	SP	HT	SI	BL	K
GB	LV	LU	LI	ST	SP	TW	GB	LV	LU	LI	ST

☯

LV	LV	LV	LV	LV	LV	GB	GB	GB	GB	GB	GB
SI	BL	K	P	TW	GB	HT	SI	BL	K	P	TW
LU	LI	ST	SP	HT	SI	LV	LU	LI	ST	SP	HT

—pattern

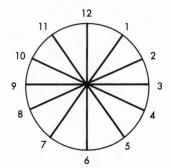

There is one level to this pattern, and as it happens, it is an interchange between a Yin parent and Yang child or a Yang parent and Yin child and vice versa:

LU	LI	ST	SP	HT	SI	BL	K	P	TW	GB	LV
BL	K	P	TW	GB	LV	LU	LI	ST	SP	HT	SI

◿ pattern

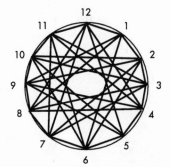

There is one level to this pattern:

LU	LI	ST	SP	HT	SI	BL	K	P	TW	GB	LV
K	P	TW	GB	LV	LU	LI	ST	SP	HT	SI	BL
LV	LU	LI	ST	SP	HT	SI	BL	K	P	TW	GB

Part Six

Additional Tools for Healing

28

intuition: your most powerful ally

"FEMININE INTUITION" IS SOMETHING THAT WOMEN ARE famous for—knowing and seeing without apparent effort. Clairvoyant or clairaudient women were burned at the stake at one time. Now such gifts are a bit more modern and acceptable. We all get that "hunch," that gut-feeling that encourages us to follow our instinct. If you're in business, maybe you've had to deal with a contract that didn't "feel right." If you're a mom, your "radar" has probably prompted you to make a sudden dash for the bathroom, where your toddler is standing on the edge of the sink, just starting to reach for the medicine cabinet. This is your intuition at work.

How does this gut-level knowledge help you in everyday life? What if you find yourself with a very strong feeling that your partner is being unfaithful? Look at that feeling. Where is the feeling in your body? Is the uncomfortable sensation right in the center of your gut, your navel area? Is it near your heart? These are the areas where your intuitive knowing physically registers its "knowing" as a tangible feeling. In meditation, this area is called your "center," a place of focus.

Be very careful to listen to such feelings and signals, and acknowledge them. To simply push them aside as suspicious, paranoid thinking will be of no help to you. Maybe that's the case, but never automatically jump to that conclusion. Treat the combined feeling and physical "symptoms" of the situation as an intuitive learning experience.

Begin to trust your gut feelings. Cultivate your intuition. Look inward to self-understanding and become your own best friend. Listen to the stillness within you, build up your inner knowing, and let it evolve into a powerful resource that you can rely on in difficult moments. Each time you acknowledge your intuition, you strengthen it. In time, it will become a sturdy ally. Should you make that investment? Which school should your child attend? Vacation this month or next? Listen for the answer in your gut.

Are you in a bad relationship? If so, what are you learning from it? How badly were you treated as a child and how much continued emotional or physical abuse will you endure as an adult? Abuse that is unchecked will never stop. Do you even recognize it as abuse? Have you re-created your childhood in your relationship? Are you ready to learn about your own patterns and how to change them?

If you are in an abusive relationship it may be because you were programmed, from childhood, to see abuse as normal. By being in it again, you have a chance to free yourself from that type of patterning for all time. Work on your own core issues without self-judgment. When you judge yourself, the inner beating you give yourself causes enormous stress.

Each time you deny your intuitive function—that little voice within that gives you "hunches"—you weaken it. Never ignore your gut feelings. How do you begin to cultivate your intuition? By listening to it when it sends you messages. And by listening, your intuition will guide you with advice on your relationship, or your work—whatever—it will silently teach you what you need to do.

Have you ever been about to drive off somewhere, perhaps for an appointment, and for no logical reason felt that you had to go back into the house for something? You know it will make you late, yet you go back in anyway? You enter, the telephone rings, you have a conversation with a friend, which delays you by five or ten minutes. You return to your car, drive off down the highway and see a tragic car accident that you could have been part of, had you not gone back into the house.

That was your intuition delaying you by those five or ten minutes. This is the part of us that can plug into the future, ten minutes ahead in time, a week, a month, or years.

Now, do you remember what the feeling felt like, when you got the urge to go back inside? Was it a sense of calm that is hard to describe, yet different from the calm of looking out onto a beautiful sunset? Or was it a more urgent pull, like you had left something boiling on the stove? Where was that feeling located? In the area near your navel? Between your navel and your heart? The center of your body? Did your stomach go into a knot? Did you feel slightly queasy or ill? Did the hairs stand up on the back of your neck, or perhaps your arms? Did you see a quick video-like picture in your mind (eidetic imagery)? These are all ways intuition manifests physically.

What organs do you think are involved in the intuitive function? Look at Liver (which houses the Soul), Kidney (which registers fear), and Heart (where spirit energy dwells).

When a fast thought, a realization, comes into your mind, and is accompanied by one or more of these feelings, recognize it as your intuition. If you have to think about it, that is your rational mind. The conscious rational mind and negative emotions—fear, paranoia—are the biggest negators of intuition.

By now you should have figured out that intuition, gut hunches, flying by the seat of your pants, clairvoyance, and psychic knowing are all one and the same. Or are they? Remember that there is a fine line between intuitive caution, and fear and paranoia. If you are continually wrong with your hunches, then you really must honestly address your own fears.

It's also important that you trust your own hunches instead

of someone else's. There are numerous people who are addicted to their psychic advisors—who are never right—and this
bothers me; both the addiction and the continued wrong
advice.

Sometimes being intuitive is hard, especially when information offered is refused and unheard, and silence is often the
only answer. As Einstein understood it, somewhere in time, the
Battle of 1066 in England has yet to be won. After a while, "I-
told-you-so" loses its gusto. And sometimes when you know
that what you have "seen" must be acted upon, yet not said,
there are ways of doing just that.

Have you ever had a dream that felt like precognition?
We've all had the experience of déjà vu—of remembering an
experience from "before" while we're in the experience. The
"before" is quite often a dream you've had, and have forgot-
ten. One such dream I had came to me on Christmas Eve
when I was a teenager. My family had gone to Connecticut to
spend Christmas with my aunt.

I awoke feeling violently nauseated. I had dreamed that
the house had caught fire and we were all severely burned or
killed. I awoke knowing it was going to happen Christmas
morning, that morning. There had been times in my childhood when my parents were not interested in listening to me
and my dreams. I knew this would be one of them. "Good
morning everyone, Merry Christmas, let's get out of the house
because it's going to go up in flames!" would not have been
well received. What to do became an instant obsession. We had
all been awake for about half an hour, my mother and aunt
were busying themselves in the kitchen preparing the turkey
and the electricity went off. My nausea—my "gut" feeling—
became worse. The electricity would somehow be connected
with the fire.

I knew I had to get everyone out of the house. So I
became an instant demanding brat. I insisted on going out for

breakfast—I was *hungry*, I whined, I wanted food; no I would *not* wait until the electricity came back on, I wanted food *now.*

This behavior was so uncharacteristic of me that within fifteen minutes everyone was dressed and bundled for a snow bound outing. We had a great Christmas brunch and drove back home about three hours later. As my aunt opened the front door, thick black smoke billowed out.

The electrical supply for the *entire* three hundred condo village malfunctioned and came in as a power surge through my aunt's heating and electrical system. It came down the kitchen stove exhaust extractor and was so intense that it cooked the thawed turkey sitting on the kitchen table. My mother and aunt would also have been nuked. It came up the heating duct next to my bed, which was fried to a crisp. It blasted out of the power outlet in the guest bathroom where my dad would have been standing doing his morning shaving ritual.

How do you develop and strengthen your intuition? The best way is through meditation. There is a gentle exercise which you can do to increase your sensitivity. It is best done while relaxed and lying down. Or you can sit in a comfortable meditation pose if you prefer. Close your eyes and focus your attention in the middle of your forehead. You do not physically look to the middle of your forehead with your eyes because if you did, you would be cross-eyed, and you would be quite uncomfortable. Your closed eyes will encounter blackness. Focus your attention and "stare" into this blackness, look into the center and go deeper and deeper into the darkness until you encounter its core. In this core there are colors that fold in and out of each other, similar to a bright tie-dye T-shirt.

As you encounter the colors, watch them as they smoothly expand within your head. I used to love doing this exercise as a child. I still do. When I close my eyes there is a wonderful round blue ball of color which is motionless, then it begins to spread and fold in on itself, and it merges into purple and white, and sometimes pinks and the hues of a beautiful sunset. As I am watching the colors, I get to a point where I'm aware that all there is is color, it has become a meditation. My mind is still and blank. There are no worries, no thoughts at all and I am completely relaxed. I find that this simple exercise helps to keep my intuition in "good shape," sort of like lifting weights or any other type of physical exercise for the body. And, as discussed in the next chapter on acupressure and auricular therapy, I wear earrings in my psychic ear point, which enhances this ability as well.

29

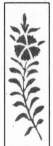

acupressure
and auricular
therapy

ACUPRESSURE OF THE EAR, OR AURICULAR THERAPY, IS A
specialized branch of what I call acu-healing or acu-therapy. It
is a branch of Oriental medicine that deals only with energy
points located on the front and back of the external ear (auricle). There are literally hundreds of very tiny points for the different organs, the limbs, mouth, the spine, sexual organs,
toothache, asthma, emotional points for happiness, for anesthesia, and the intuitive—you name it, it's there. These points are
pressed with a small hand-held tool or instrument having solid
gold and silver ends, connected by any organic substance. Don't
use metal. My favorite tool's rod is carved from thirty-thousand
year old fossilized mastodon bone. Points can be worked to stop
smoking, as well as drug and alcohol addiction. More than
2,000 years ago, in the *Nei Ching,* Ling Shu said "The ear is the
place where all the channels meet."

In my work, I have found that by going straight to an
organ point on the ear—rather than working a series of points
along the organ energy flow on the body—the beneficial
results are faster, greater, and far outweigh those of bodywork,
although, as with anything, results vary from individual to
individual.

Clients usually drift into a state of altered consciousness, similar to sleep, in which they release old emotional problems and trauma from childhood and from what appears to be (depending upon your belief system) "past lives" or "ancestor memory." Sometimes the client will talk with the voice of her four-year-old childself and actually exude smells from her past surroundings that have been trapped in body memory.

In one particular case, a client gave off a distinct smell of clover as she described, in her little girl's voice, how she loved to run into a field, behind the family home, throw herself into the clover face down and breathe in its scent. A little later in her story, the smell became that of fresh paint.

In the session, she described her day of play with her little red-haired friend Mary, which included lying in the clover and then later, playing jacks on the steps of her newly painted porch. She neither liked the smell of the paint, nor the color change, and was most indignant about the entire situation, especially that no one had consulted her. After a pause, she said, "Well, I am only a child, so why should they?" She talked about her daily routine of sitting on the porch steps at the end of the day to wait for her father's return from work. On this particular day, her dad failed to return from the city. While at his office he suffered a massive stroke, died, and never walked up those steps or into her life again.

She cried softly as she "slept," and awoke wondering why she was crying. I told her, word for word, her account of that day. Finally, she understood that she had never recovered from the trauma of her father's death and had carried the pain and grief for seventy-one years. She never understood why she became so violently ill around newly painted places, or why the smell of fresh paint frightened her so. In this three-hour session, she also came to terms with guilt she felt when her mother died from cancer while she was away at college. At the end of the session, she looked twenty years younger. At eighty, she has still maintained the age loss that's accompanied ridding herself of the pain and guilt attached to her parents' deaths.

This work is very interesting for me because I never know how a session will go. I often find myself working points that were not called for after taking the pulses, and it is these points, worked intuitively, that often generate the most unexpected and dramatic healings. As negative energy is drawn from a client's body, I will sometimes see scenes from their childhood, or past lives, or ancestor memory situations that are causing present day problems. My body temperature rises, pain will be present in my body where pain has gone from the client's, and this is sometimes accompanied by nausea.

During one session my hands became so full of someone's painful energy that I had to excuse myself to place my hands in a nearby bowl of water. Water draws out negative energy and this water promptly turned dark gray while the client stared in disbelief and remarked "That came out of me? Good gracious!"

During another session, while sitting outside on a lawn, giving an impromptu neck massage to someone with very bad arthritis pain, my hands became crippled and gnarled and bore no resemblance to my normal fingers. I was unable to straighten them, and it was actually the client who suggested that I drive my fingers into the grass and soil to "earth" the negative energy I had drawn from his body.

One of the most interesting cases I was sent was a man in his early forties who was in terrible shape from everything you could possibly imagine. He was overweight by about 150 pounds, and he looked at least sixty years old. He was an alcoholic with severe liver and kidney damage, and he suffered from the chronic pain and fever that accompanies kidney disease. He smoked four packs of cigarettes a day. He had been to specialists all over the world for tests and hormone treatments to try to achieve a normal sperm count—his wife was longing for a child. He had repeatedly been told that his low sperm count was linked to his smoking and drinking, yet he could not give up these addictions, and even short periods of abstinence had failed to help the sperm situation. That is why he had been sent to me, to do anti-smoking and anti-drinking work. It wasn't until the end of the session that he told me about his sperm count problem.

As I worked his various ear points, the energy coming out of him was so toxic that at one point I felt as if I would black out; at another point I felt quite drunk. When I worked his various Lung points from the deep lung bronchioles through the upper lung area, the nausea I felt was indescribable. He did the deep breathing exercises that I managed to live through. Then, for no conscious reason, my tool went to the point for his prostate gland. The burst of blocked energy was so great my hand was thrown off his ear. By this time he was snoring, worn out from the breathing exercises, and awoke to a most unladylike exclamation as I tried to regain my composure. Energy continued to release until the point was quite clear and the tiny tool seemed to weigh fifteen pounds. At the end of the session, his temperature had vanished and he said he felt like a "new man." Three days later, he came back for another treatment and although he had no desire to smoke or drink, we did a bit more lung work. A week later he returned, having already lost ten pounds, to announce jubilantly that for the first time in his life he had a normal sperm count.

In ancient China, as a result of acupuncture of the ear, earrings came into being for health purposes rather than for our modern-day decorative purposes. Even Hippocrates and Galen of Greece, around 470 B.C., wrote of ear piercing and earring wearing to relieve and treat menstrual problems.

In these ancient times, if an organ was low in energy, gold earrings would be placed in a pierced acu-point for stimulation; silver earrings if the organ had too much energy. Gemstones were added for their therapeutic effects; for example, emerald would be worn to prevent miscarriage and aid in childbirth; amethyst to purify Blood; ruby to regulate menstruation and enhance fertility; and citrine to boost sexual energy, and strengthen Kidney and Liver. These benefits were then trans-

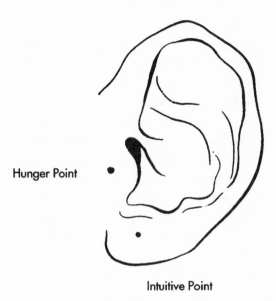

Hunger Point

Intuitive Point

mitted through the gold or silver. The traditional modern-day point for ear piercing is in the middle of the fleshy lobe. This is the intuitive, third eye, or psychic point. It is important that gold rather than silver be worn here. Gold, combined with an amethyst or emerald, which are both traditionally regarded as very spiritual stones, will have an added positive effect on the intuitive function.

The ancients treated diseases of the feminine Yin organs via earrings in the left ear and diseases of the male Yang organs would similarly be treated via the right ear. Left side, feminine side, right side, male side. For some situations, the left ear is considered more powerful than the right ear for balancing energy because the left side is the feminine, receptive side of the body. I normally take into account whether someone is right- or left-handed. A right-handed individual will get more benefit from work on the right ear.

One good example of auricular therapy at work in modern times is the recent interest in "staples" in the ear for weight-loss purposes. There is a point on the ear known as the "Hunger Point," and this point can be worked to help someone if they wish to change their diet for weight loss or weight gain. Working the Hunger Point helps to curb or enhance the appetite and is particularly beneficial for energetically balancing bulimic or anorexic clients.

Would we all have more sexual energy and balance if we pierced our noses in the traditional East Indian point? The nose piercing spot is the Stomach acupuncture point. Stomach is an Earth organ. The ancients always began treatment with Earth organs. The Earth organ pair is Stomach and Spleen. Stomach is Yang, or male, and gives energy to Spleen, which is Yin—and vice versa, a harmonious flow between the two. In energetic terms, Spleen governs the sexual organs; physically, it cleans the blood by removing dead red cells and makes B cells which make antibodies that fight disease. We know gold stimulates a point (brings in energy) and silver sedates (releases excess energy). Gold is Yang metal, silver Yin. Nose piercing is always on the Yin (left) side, with a gold nose ring or stud. So, a pierced nose will constantly be stimulating Stomach, which will always have plenty of energy to give to partner Spleen, which equals good sex drive, good reproductive system, good immune system.

Similarly, in ancient times, gold bands were worn around wrists to regulate and stimulate all the organ pulses. Gold belts were worn around the waist area for the same reason, drawing in the Sun's healing energy. It was believed that gemstones gently pulled in the energy from the planets that governed them, planets also associated with the Five Elements and the individual organs.

Throughout the ancient worlds, craftspeople created talismanic jewelry for protection, healing, and optimum health. Different cultures in different lands appear to have shared one basic knowledge.

30

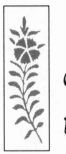

color
therapy

EACH OF THE FIVE ELEMENTS, AND HENCE EACH ORGAN PAIR, is associated with a color. The color for Earth is yellow, Metal is white, Water, blue or black, Wood is green, and Fire is red.

Generally, in day-to-day living, we pay little attention to color. Colors are just "there," around us in nature, at work, in our homes, and in our closets and drawers. However, if we begin to observe colors more closely, the ones we like, the ones we dislike, we can begin to learn details about our inner workings that may surprise us and shed light on our physical and emotional health. It is useful to keep the colors of the Five Elements in mind for color therapy purposes, and to really listen to what your intuitive and unconscious is trying to tell you on a daily basis.

What color underwear were you attracted to this morning? Did you *feel* like wearing something blue to work but *decided* to wear green instead—mind overriding intuition—and then came home a great deal more weary than normal and definitely not in the mood for sex?

Perhaps your Water energy was low, and it was trying to "tell" you that it needed the color energy boost from the blue. Because Kidney is the storehouse for all energy, when it becomes depleted, the Spleen energy is the next energy to go.

The sexual organs, sexual energy, and desire are governed by Spleen. When you decided to wear green, the color associated with the element Wood, green only gave further energy to Wood and depleted Water even more, which then pulled energy from Earth.

One of the most profound color experiences I have had took place in Chicago's O'Hare Airport. Between terminals there is an underground connecting tunnel with a moving walkway. The walls of the tunnel are paneled with squares of soft pastel shades covering the entire color spectrum. Overhead, there are bright neon lights in the colors of the rainbow, ending at the far end with bright white light. Bright colors are considered Yang, and pastel shades are Yin.

On that particular day I was wearing black. Black is black because it contains all of the other colors, or absorbs all other colors. White reflects all colors. Just by wearing black, the therapeutic effects of every color in the tunnel were being pulled into my body's energy system, and by the time the moving walkway had reached the white light and I was stepping into the other terminal, I was feeling extremely calm, almost as if I had been cleansed in some manner, or had undergone a mini-massage session. Everyone passing through that airport tunnel was affected by those colors, whether they consciously were aware of it is another matter. Learn to be sensitive to how colors affect you.

Dr. Norman Shealy[1] of Springfield, Missouri—a noted neurosurgeon—has a healing facility in Springfield. One of his treatment methods involves using sequenced flashing colored lights, which balance the neurochemistry in the brain. He works with patients who have chronic pain, depression, sleep disorders, and other assorted problems. As a Diagnostic Intuitive (meaning intuition figures largely in my healing work), I stud-

1. Shealy Institute, 1328 East Evergreen, Springfield, Missouri 65803.

ied the *science* of intuition with him at this facility and found his methods to be fascinating. In many hospitals across the contry, leading surgeons are working with intuitive diagnosticians who mentally scan the body for illness and disease. It is now possible to aquire a Ph.D. in this field of study.

The importance of color, color therapy, and using color for healing is hardly new. Color has been used by many cultures for hundreds of years. When people are in mourning it is customary to wear either black or white. Wearing white assists in clearing grief from the lungs. Wearing black helps to clear grief from the lungs because of Kidney's "pull" effect over Lung. Wearing black also helps to gain back general energy that has been lost through the emotional strain of the grieving process.

If I know a client is coming to me for a specific problem, I will put colored sheets on my therapy table according to the client's needs. A client made a booking for a session one day and said that she was very tired, that she had some kidney pain, maybe a bladder infection coming on, and was "miserable." The color for the Water element—Kidney and Bladder—is blue, so I put a dark blue towel over the table for her to lie on. Upon her arrival, I gave her a cup of cinnamon and cranberry leaf tea—cinnamon has a warming effect on the kidneys, cranberry flushes out in an alkaline manner—took her pulses and found the following: Bladder was low, Kidney excessive, and Lung and Large Intestine were also low in energy.

As soon as I began massaging her upper back, shoulders, and neck area in preparation for her auricular therapy session, she started to cry and eventually laughed a great deal, saying "I feel great, and you haven't really started yet!"

I worked the client's appropriate ear points for the organs involved, plus other points for additional problems she was having. She released a great deal of old, stale, blocked energy. By "released," I mean that I could feel a very slight pulsing or buzzing sensation flowing into my fingers. All her kidney pain was gone fifteen minutes into the session. We sat talking for a while after her visit, going over issues that had come up.

When I went to remove the dark blue towel she had been lying on, I discovered the area of the towel that had been beneath her right kidney was quite hot—twenty minutes after her getting off the table—and that the rest of the towel was cold. It is interesting because when she called to say she had "kidney pain," I assumed she meant both kidneys, but it had only been the right kidney that was bothering her. She was just as surprised as I was. It was apparent that the blue color had helped to pull whatever negative energy was affecting her kidney, out of her body.

All my life, as far back as I can remember, I have loathed the color red. Red was my mother's favorite color and, consequently, her choice for a lot of my dresses. I never understood why I disliked the color because I quite enjoyed seeing red worn by others. But I would recoil when she tried to put me in my little red velvet dress and matching shoes. I also disliked yellow. Years later, I came to realize that, as a sexually abused child, the last thing my unconscious would have wanted to deal with was a color that actually gave energy to my sexual area. Red, the color of the Fire Element, gives energy to Earth, associated with yellow, the color of the organ flow that governs sexuality, the Spleen organ flow.

A skeptic would say that is all too pat. But it isn't because I've had similar situations happen to me all my life. Everyone has heard of the familiar expressions involving colors.

Now consider such expressions in relation to the Five Element Theory.

"Feeling blue?" Maybe you're so depressed that Heart energy is pulling energy from Kidney.

"Green with envy?" Perhaps you are so full of jealousy and envy that your Lung is pulling from Liver.

"White as a sheet?" Perhaps you've just had such a shock that your Heart is pulling energy from Lung.

"Yellow-bellied coward?" Perhaps you are so timid and

afraid of a situation that your Kidney is pulling energy from your Spleen.

Or do you remember the groundbreaking Swedish film "I Am Curious Yellow"? It was about sexual awakening.

So mad you just "saw red?" Perhaps you are so furious with someone that your Liver is pulling energy from your Heart.

"In a black mood?" So mad that your Liver is pulling energy from Kidney.

"In a fog?" So confused and full of self-doubt that you don't know what to do and become despondent as your Heart pulls energy from your Lungs.

A negative emotion that begins in one organ, if not addressed, if not dealt with, if not acknowledged, if not accepted by oneself or a partner ("Listen to what I'm saying, please!"), gets worse and goes to a deeper level in another organ.

As you can begin to see, Five Element thinking will support you in living your life in a more healthy way. Until I began

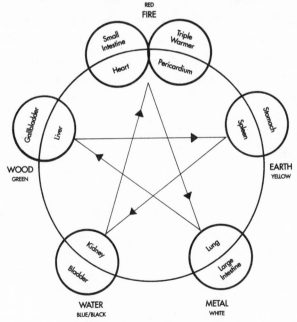

Five Elements color associations

this work, I had never dreamed that my reluctance to wear the color yellow had a sexual basis and that red, associated with Fire, could have actually helped return energy to areas of sexual abuse, and that the Spleen-governed sexual organs could have benefited from the regenerative powers of Earth's color, yellow.

When I decided to heal my sexual abuse memories, I happened to be back in Bermuda after some extensive traveling, and the first thing I did was paint my bathroom Chinese Red. I purchased red candles that would burn for seven days, and, as I lit a candle, I would pray for healing and help with my process of facing and letting go of the memories. Then I began taking hot baths in the dark, with only one red candle burning, with jasmine, lavender, and rosemary oils, and ten pounds of Epsom salts in the water. And I would concentrate on my memories of sexual abuse in this atmosphere of healing water, warmth, aromatherapy oils, and light. With each bath the terrible pictures in my mind disappeared down the drain until I could "look" at them, lecture, or speak about them without any emotion, fear, or terror. When I'd finally dealt with the abuse—the emotions and the memories—once and for all, many aspects of my life began to change. I began to open up and be less fearful all around. I felt lighter, looked better, and smiled a lot more for no particular reason. I did these baths three times a week for ten months. My bathroom is still painted red, but now a bubble bath is just that, a bubble bath, and there are no ghosts in the water with me.

3 I

healing anger

NEGATIVE EMOTIONS, WHEN ALLOWED TO GO UNATTENDED, WILL fester. Anger has been implicated by researchers in depression, high blood pressure, heart disease, arthritis, stress, substance abuse, and obesity. Women of extremes—who either inhibit or vent their anger—have higher rates of breast cancer.[1]

That does not mean that it is inappropriate to feel anger. There are situations in everyday life where it is appropriate. What is important is really feeling that anger, connecting with it, and allowing yourself to be angry, and then be done with it. Does the anger that you are experiencing in the present time really have its roots earlier on in life? Perhaps then, a similar situation arose and the person with whom you are dealing "now" is really receiving the brunt of anger that, in reality, perhaps belonged, say, to your mother or father when you were six or sixteen? Is it simply a similar situation with another person pushing your buttons?

As I've progressed with my own healing and dealt with childhood issues, I've noticed something quite surprising, and at the same time healing. At one time, I would get angry at some-

1. Denis Foley and Eileen Nechas, *Women's Encyclopedia of Health and Emotional Healing* (Emmaus, PA: Rodale Press, 1993), p. 14.

thing or someone and "stew" internally, gnashing my teeth (anger can manifest in teeth problems) for a few hours, thirty minutes, or a twenty-mile drive. I now find that I'm mad for maybe a minute and then it's gone completely. Sometimes in fact, the anger lasts for a few seconds. Sometimes there is no anger at all.

However, if I become angry, I will quietly study the situation in my mind, and ask myself, "Apart from anger, is there anything else you feel? Have you felt like this before, and if so, when?" What will happen is that a memory may pop up from ages past, when for example I was twenty, and I'll remember a whole specific situation in great detail, feel it, understand it, and let it go, then ask myself, "Was there a time before that?"

By the time I am finished, I am looking at a time when I was three years old, and I have released excessive "now" time anger that really began when someone ignored me when I was very small or implied I was stupid or laughed at me in an unkind manner or didn't believe me or listen to me. This process has taken perhaps two or three minutes, maybe less than that, because "time," as we know it, does not exist in the mind.

This method of back-track healing (my label for it) was developed by Dan Jones, Ph.D., and John Lee, author of numerous books, including *The Flying Boy: Healing the Wounded Man* and *Recovery Plain and Simple*. John calls this method PEER™ Therapy, which stands for Primary Emotional Energy Recovery. I have trained in PEER Therapy and have found it to be one of the fastest methods for removing old "garbage" emotions from body memory for myself and clients.

I want to heal all my childhood issues, and no longer be trapped in the person my childhood created from abuse and dysfunction. That desire to heal is so intense that I push myself to look at issues that are difficult to confront. It is scary; however, I have lost the desire and the patience to sit on a therapist's couch talking about the same issue week after week.

That is far from healing as far as I am concerned. It is living in a state of "wound." Sharing talk of wounds, living endlessly in support groups, bonding by reason of pain and trauma are ways of existing that hardly help one expand beyond the past. Want to stay in the past where it is now "safe" because you finally know what happened to you? Then stay in a support group. But that's really the last place you should want to be if you're really healing the past after you have faced the reality of who and what and why you are "you."

Face the fear and the panic just once instead of running to your support group, and you've already begun to reprogram yourself—your brain—for more than just survival in groups, which is far from really living.

You were abused? Okay, recognize your patterns. Take the time to list all your problem areas: work, people, the kids, sex, elevators, relationships, intimacy, dark rooms, food, stealing, compulsive lying, alcohol, *et cetera*. The aim of this exercise is to get on with life and consciously stop the old patterns. You're afraid of heights? Because someone held you out of a window as a child? Fine, look down through closed windows in tall buildings until the fear vanishes and you become interested in the tiny cars, people, and events below. Elevators or dark places terrify you because you were shut in a tightly packed closet as a child? Then ride crowded elevators until the fear passes and the people, their perfume, their clothes, faces, their shapes are what fascinates you. Even if you can't recall the old memory, the old reason for the fear and anger, confront it anyway.

Take a fear and make it a meditation. A meditation you'll master in twenty-four or forty-eight hours. Just do it. You will feel good about yourself and the process. If I can do it—and as a child, I was dangled off the edge of a boat so I would cooperate with my sexual abuser—then you can too. Anything less is hiding behind your momma's skirt, and not really living.

I want active tools that I can take home and use so that fear of abandonment, emotional abuse, fear of engulfment—*et cetera, et cetera ad infinitum*—cease to be my bedfellows and work partners for the rest of my life.

Be careful to avoid letting anger progress into bitterness and resentment. You will ultimately end up brooding over it. Which is the same as saying, don't let the anger sit in the Liver and then spread to the Spleen. This negative, anger-generated-energy will affect your sexuality and your immune system, because that is what Spleen takes care of physically—the immune defense system—and you will give off a wall of feelings that will be so thick no one will want to get anywhere near you. Stop your negative emotions before they disease their way out of your body.

32

visualization and meditation

SOME YEARS AGO I MET A MAN WHO SHARED A USEFUL VISUALization technique with me, and I want to share it with you.

At the time, I had been experiencing discomfort in my lower left abdomen, and, having previously undergone surgery on my left ovary for the removal of a cyst, I wondered if I had somehow strained the scar tissue. A visit to my doctor and a sonogram revealed that another cyst or tumor had grown in the same area. My left ovary was the only ovary I had left. My doctor is a wonderful, gentle man, a gynecologist who specializes in infertility and microsurgery. He told me that because of my previous surgeries in the pelvic area, he might not be able to save my one remaining ovary. He let me know that I might even be facing a hysterectomy. He asked me to come back on Tuesday for a pre-op sonogram. It was during my divorce. I was thirty-four years old.

My entire body went numb; every cell froze as I realized that I was facing radical surgery. At that time in my life, all I could think of were my three, once female, cats. Would I, too, become an "it"? It was a Friday. Once again the passage of time had given me a grace period.

On Saturday I went to a party, not for the cheer, but

because I wanted to get drunk in the safety of a friend's house, a friend who made the best Bloody Marys on the island. I wanted to drown my sorrows. Drinking was not something I indulged in; having been a kidney patient for so many years, alcohol was strictly taboo for me. Yet that night I didn't care much about my kidneys.

Almost as soon as I arrived, and while I was in the middle of my first Bloody Mary, a man approached me and we began to talk. I'd never seen him before, which is pretty hard when you live on a nineteen-mile-long island. But there was something familiar about him; his shoulder-length, wavy brown hair and kind eyes, marvelous laugh, and warm handshake made me feel very comfortable. So we settled in to talk our way through the night. We were still there, along with about ten other people, at sunrise for the traditional Sunday morning breakfast of codfish and potatoes served with tomatoes, avocado, boiled egg, and banana, a Bermudian tradition that goes back to the 1600s.

The stranger had shared with me his interests in nutrition, fasting, and yoga, told me that he ate fish and chicken sparingly, never red meat or pork. He was actually mostly vegetarian and from what he said, I gathered he didn't need to eat that much. We seemed alike in many ways. I enjoyed his company, and his similar thoughts about life and daily living reminded me of a friend I'd had as a child, a friend who had given me a code to live by when I was four.

He eventually asked me why there was so much sadness in my eyes, sadness my smile couldn't cover. So I told him about my impending surgery. He asked me if I had ever "visualized" during meditation. I replied that I didn't know what visualization was.

He asked if I had ever tried to imagine myself surrounded by protective golden light. I had tried the technique but could not seem to master it. I always asked God to surround me in protective golden light but could never pretend to see it all around me. So he asked if I had a particular connection with any powerful animals. Yes, I did, there was a black panther I regularly dreamed about since the night of my thirteenth birthday. So he told me what to do.

"Go home and have a warm Epsom salt bath, about eight pounds for your body weight,[1] and then get comfortable in something warm, somewhere you can meditate. Close your eyes and feel all the parts of your body, starting with your feet and working your way up to the top of your head. Feel the breath going in and out of your nose. Feel your heart beat. Feel the relaxed state of your body. If there is pain, feel it, melt into it, do not be afraid of it. When you are relaxed and comfortable, imagine that your panther has become very small and has entered your body where the cyst is located. The panther will shred the growth, eat every inch of it, and lick the whole area clean of anything that does not belong there."

It was already morning, so I went home, had the bath, put on my woolly footed pajamas and snuggled myself into bed to do the meditation the stranger taught me. At one point during the visualization it seemed as if the whole situation was quite out of control: the panther was shredding my cyst and surrounding area so ferociously that it frightened me. I had this odd notion that opening my eyes would not be something I would relish, in case I really was shredded—that's how real the imagined visualization became, I was not controlling it, it was going on all by itself, as if a dream was running inside my entire body. My heart was pounding with fright. When I finally mustered up the courage to open my eyes and look down at my tummy, the house was in darkness and I couldn't see a thing. Clasping my pelvic region, to hold it together in case it was shredded (which sounds ridiculous now, but you had to be there to appreciate the intensity of it all), I climbed out of bed

---

1. One note of caution: if you wish to do this meditation, hot baths are not recommended for those who are pregnant, have heart problems, high blood pressure, or diabetes. Some people have also been known to become dizzy if not accustomed to hot baths.

and turned on the light. It was 9 P.M. I had been meditating for over twelve hours and it had seemed like no more than an hour or two at the most. To my relief, I was intact.

When I returned to the hospital on Tuesday for the pre-op sonogram, there was no growth; it had vanished over the weekend.

33

diet and fasting

THE FLOW OF ENERGY IN YOUR BODY MEANS NOTHING IF your whole system is malnourished! In 1992, *Time* magazine ran an article on health care and revealed that, due to the spiraling costs involved in Western medical care (which consists mainly of expensive tests, drugs, and surgery), the National Institute of Health in America budgeted $2 million received from Congress to look into alternative and energetic medical methods for healing. The Institute was inspired by reports such as those from Dr. Dean Ornish of the University of California at San Francisco who estimated that half of the $12 billion spent on heart bypass surgery in 1990 could have been eliminated if the patients had changed their diets, stopped smoking, and had done relaxation exercises.

When considering your overall diet, it is important to eat sufficient protein, fiber, carbohydrates, and fat on a daily basis. Food sources high in fiber are beans, potatoes, broccoli, brussels sprouts, carrots, turnips, eggplant, brown rice, shredded wheat type cereals, corn, pears, and blueberries. Protein is found in all meats and fish (especially herrings and sardines), dairy products, eggs, beans, and tofu. For women who are menopausal, good sources of calcium are to be found in milk, cheese, yogurt, okra, turnip greens, broccoli, nuts, bok choy, mustard greens, kale, oysters, sardines, and salmon.

The diet I now follow grew out of my need to heal the chronic bladder infections and progressive kidney disease that had plagued me most of my life. After laser surgery on my left kidney, I dropped certain foods from my diet; foods that are known to produce oxalic acid kidney stones as a by-product of their digestion. This diet also happens to benefit women who suffer from yeast infections because many of these same foods also promote the growth of yeast (*Candida albicans*) bacteria.

Yeast infections often occur as a side effect while taking antibiotics—which destroy friendly as well as harmful bacteria—and in women this side effect shows up mostly in the vaginal area. Some women, for no apparent reason, are plagued by yeast infections throughout their lives.

The following dietary changes were given to me by the Lahey Clinic in Burlington, Massachusetts, after my surgery— the idea being that these changes would prevent new kidney stones from developing. For two years I religiously followed this diet and found that all of the small kidney stones that were not removed, dissolved on their own. At the age of thirty-three, for the first time in my life, I no longer suffered from bladder and kidney problems or infections. The surgeon also recommended that I drink eight 8 oz. glasses of water a day, however this was too much water for my 105-pound body. Generally, I drink about four glasses a day. You just have to use your own judgment on this—"one-size dose" does not fit everyone! These dietary changes also help to overcome Candida problems.

Foods to be eliminated:

Try to eliminate the following foods: sugars, honey, maple syrup, molasses, junk foods (i.e. chips, cheese doodles, most fast foods, etc.), soda pop—especially root beer (hard on the kidneys)—cider, apple, grape, and tomato juices; ice cream, caffeinated tea and coffee, wine, alcohol, beer, mineral water, peanuts and peanut butter, pineapple, chocolate and hot chocolate, spinach, beets, rhubarb, cheese, milk, vinegar, sour cream, mushrooms, malted foods, commercially dried fruits, breads and cookies with yeast, pork, lamb, all red meats, and fried foods. Never consume saccharine or aspartame—both are laboratory synthesized chemicals, and the former has been linked to bladder cancer in laboratory rats who were unfortunate enough to be fed massive doses of it. Learn to enjoy the real taste of foods without adding any kind of sweetener and this will also cut down on PMS problems.

One of the reasons why it is so important to eliminate sugars from your diet is because Candida (yeast) thrives on sugar. And, from information compiled by Gaston Naessens of Canada, we know that "tumor cells utilize the energy produced by the destruction of carbohydrates for the synthesis of cellular proteins at greater levels than normal cells."[1] Or simply put, cancer cells pig out on sugars, which gives them enormous energy to really gorge on body protein and multiply like crazy.

Foods that are allowed:

Chicken and fish, each only once a week (3 oz. per serving, maximum 9 oz. per week, allowing for cheating). I do not eat fried foods, except stir-fried dishes prepared in very good quality oil, such as olive, peanut, or sunflower oils. I also eat bananas, pears, and apples, eggs (three a week), rice (I like white Jasmine from Thailand, and wild rice or brown rice. Don't go for the packaged processed rices—most of the nutrients have been stripped), corn and corn products, buckwheat, oatmeal, all kinds of beans, yogurt, all vegetables except those listed above. These days I am reluctant to eat fish, (especially the bottom feeders

---

1. From a brochure published by Gaston Naessens regarding the treatment of cancer.

and shell fish). With the increasing pollution of the earth's oceans, who knows if the fish came from a toxin-free area? I also feel it is important to eat raw garlic or take garlic pills every day, along with other vitamin supplements, as well as Royal Jelly in 300 mg. capsules. Royal Jelly—albeit expensive—has proven beneficial for morning sickness during pregnancy.

Here is a list of vitamins and minerals that are crucial to anyone experiencing problems with their female system (especially Candida). These supplements are highly recommended by many sources, most notably by Bob Flaws in his book on cervical dysplasia. His recommended doses are higher than the approved RDAs, so you should check with your health care practioner for appropriate doses for you. Recommended are vitamins A, B_6, B_{12}, C, E, Folic acid, Zinc Picolinate, and Selenium.[2]

Pau D'Arco tea, from the Amazon, is reputed to be beneficial for treating both Candida and cancer.

If you have symptoms of gas and bloating, and your symptoms worsen while fasting, the cause could be yeast beasties dying in the intestines and giving off death-fume-toxins that will be absorbed into the bloodstream. Generally, drinking plenty of water is important because water flushes the system out and keeps the tissues clear. If you suffer from Candida, taking acidophilus pills orally, and acidophilus enemas and douches have also been known to help.

Many women who have vaginal yeast infections also have amoebas or *Giardia lamblia* at the same time in their intestines. Both are microscopic parasites picked up from contaminated water, improperly washed food, or passed from dirty unwashed hands of the food preparer. The presence of these organisms causes bloating, alternating diarrhea and constipation, or diar-

2. Contact Metagenics International, 971 Calle Negocia, San Clemente, CA 92629, 1-800-692-9400. Ask for Chlorotene, Intrinisi B_{12}/Folate, Multigenics, and Zinc Picolinate.

rhea, gas, food allergies, chronic fatigue, and nebulous to excruciating abdominal pain.

The reason the symptoms of *Giardia* are so confusing has to do with the lifestyle and life cycle of the *Giardia*. First of all, they are living in your small and large intestines, eating everything nutritious they can. As they digest your food, they give off gas. Quite simply, they fart. You bloat and get abdominal pain. It can be particularly painful when large numbers die off at once and give off death fumes and new ones are being born at the same time and are ravenously hungry, just like any newborn. A lot of people with so-called irritable bowel syndrome more than likely have *Giardia lamblia*. Because there are foods that irritate the *Giardia lamblia*, like garlic and onions, both containing natural antibiotics, they can actually kill off the organism. Sometimes, repeated stool testing has to be done before these little four-eyed monsters are identified. *Giardia lamblia* can be present without symptoms for years.

In my own case, I suddenly became nauseous at a dinner party, left the table, suffered instant and violent vomiting and explosive diarrhea and my abdomen ballooned so that I looked quite pregnant. All of this in the course of ten minutes. The pain was unbearable and walking was impossible. I was rushed to the hospital, my appendix removed, and there was nothing wrong with it aside from mild inflamation. Two months later, *Giardia lamblia* were finally detected in my stool by a special laboratory in Atlanta, Georgia.

Artemisia annua and *Artemisia absinthium* (commonly known as wormwood) are both known to kill off parasites. Pumpkin seeds, betel nut and meliae seeds, golden seal, citrus seed extract, and vermox are also all good for eliminating many different types of worms as well as other types of parasites.

If you are prone to bladder infections or bladder irritation—burning during and after urination, sometimes with severe irritation, as if your bladder is trying to expel itself from your body, or the feeling that you still have to "go" a few minutes after you've just "gone"—drink several glasses of non-mineral water and cranberry juice. Unsweetened cranberry juice is very helpful for cutting down the acidity in the urine. But be careful; too much cranberry juice can result in anemia, because the alkalinity inhibits the absorption of iron by the blood. The Harvard Medical School conducted a study on cranberry juice in 1991 and found that it "contains compounds that prevent microbes from clinging to the bladder wall and triggering urinary tract infections."[3] Pure essential oil of lavender (not synthetic) is also very soothing to dab right onto the genital area if the area is irritated or inflamed from a bladder infection. The essential oil (which is very strong) must first be diluted in almond oil. I use about 10-15 drops of lavender to one ounce of almond oil.

Always remember, however, that if symptoms persist for more than a few days, it is important to seek medical attention as the condition could be serious. Being afraid to find out what is wrong never made an illness or disease go away.

Many years ago, Dr. Harry Quigley, head of the Glaucoma Department at the Johns Hopkins Hospital in Baltimore, said to me, "If you want to be healthy, think poor—eat simply—grains, vegetables, and beans." It's been very good advice.

Fasting

Many cultures around the world for many centuries have believed that it is helpful to fast. Fasting means you drink only water, at least one day a week. Fasting gives the entire body a rest, and the fast is often connected with a day of prayer. But more important, fasting gives the heart time off from having to work extremely hard while pumping extra blood to the stom-

3. *American Health* magazine, June 1994, p. 10.

ach muscles during digestion. In terms of exercise, the heart works equally as hard, whether we walk a mile or eat a big meal.

When we fast, or go without solid food and drink only water, the entire digestive system starts to clear out accumulated debris that has built up over the years. Toxins, pesticides, drug residues are released into the bloodstream, from the intestines in particular, and from body tissues. This buildup can result in headaches, fevers, and muscle and joint pain. Fasting has been shown to help high blood pressure, allergies, heart disease, arthritis, depression, any inflammatory illness, and even schizophrenia.

Before going onto a pure water fast, I build up to the fast by drinking a highly nutritious vegetable drink that I developed many years ago. I do the vegetable juice pre-fast for five days because I have found that most toxins have already been released from my body by the time I get to the pure water fast program.

Here is my recipe, made from grocery store vegetables— hence the terms "bunch" of carrots or "bunch" of celery. Make sure that they have been organically grown without exposure to any pesticides or chemicals, and be sure to wash and peel them thoroughly. This recipe will yield about two quarts and will last two people two days.

FASTING JUICE

4 ripe avocados
4 ripe, bright red, large tomatoes
2 bunches of bright orange carrots
2 bunches of bright dark green celery
1 bunch of parsley
1 head of garlic
3 large yellow lemons

Optional addition every once in a while
4 large red beets

Take all the ingredients except the avocados and put them through a juicer. I find it helpful to liquefy the avocados in a blender. When you have enough liquid made from the carrots, celery, and lemons, add that to the avocados and blend. I discovered that my juicer got less clogged when I did it this way simply because the avocado mixture is very thick and would make my machine run over. Your machine may not do that. This fasting juice is loaded with vitamins and minerals, and is very nutritious, even when you are not fasting. It is great as a "zap" for low energy days, or if you have been out in a very polluted city where airborne germs and pollution are rampant.

Often I prefer to make the juice up in batches of eight glasses worth at a time. For that you would reduce the recipe to: one lemon, one avocado, six large carrots, eighteen large celery stalks, one large tomato, half a head of garlic and half a bunch of parsley.

Cold-pressed olive oil
1 tablespoon, twice daily

To keep the bowels eliminating toxic waste buildup, take the olive oil each day that you are on the vegetable juice part of the pre-fast program. Laxative teas are also helpful and can be bought from health food stores. Never take store-bought laxative medicine while on a fast.

During a pre-fast, I drink only my own vegetable juice mixture, alternating it with bottled, non-mineral water and lemon juice for at least five days. At night I drink chamomile tea before bed.

I also use enemas and colonics during a fast. Enemas cleanse the rectum or lower bowel with water, and colonic irrigation reaches farther up into the digestive tract by cleaning out the large intestine itself and breaking away deposits that may have been clinging to the intestinal walls for many years.

Colonics are gentle, beneficial, and you'll feel great after having one. They are not at all uncomfortable. Acidophilus capsules should be taken in conjunction with colonics, to restore the natural "good" bacteria of the intestines. Acidophilus can also be introduced into the lower bowel by breaking open a capsule, and including the acidophilus powder in the enema water. Be sure to use filtered, distilled, or reverse-osmosis purified water for enemas and colonics so that you do not introduce any water-borne parasites—such as *Giardia*—into your digestive system.[4]

At the end of five days of the vegetable juice (no solid food), I go onto pure bottled water with fresh lemon juice (one teaspoon per glass) added for another five days. I follow with three more days of the vegetable juice, and then simple salads and Jasmine rice from Thailand for another three days. I prefer Jasmine rice to brown rice because it has more vitamins and minerals than brown.

During the pure water cleansing fast, my energy levels are high, my thinking is clear, and I feel spiritually renewed. My morning meditations are deeper, and yoga is effortless. When breaking a cleansing fast, it is very important to come off the fast by eating only simple salads, rice, and yogurt for three days before building up to your regular diet again. I generally do this cleansing routine in the spring and autumn, and more often if I feel it's needed.

What happens if you end a fast by going straight back into normal heavy meals? You can become very ill. This happened to me the first time I took part in a fast at the Yoga Retreat on Paradise Island in the Bahamas where I was on staff many years ago. We went on a ten-day fast, going straight into water and lemon juice only. I understood the principles of going onto a fast and fasting, but no one told me how to break a fast. My first meal

---

4. A normal, healthy digestive system does not require enemas on a daily basis. Overuse of enemas can impair the natural function of the bowel.

was an enormous plate of macaroni and cheese with onions, tomatoes, and mushrooms, soybean loaf and a salad.

That night I ran a temperature of 104°F, was practically comatose, and the next morning felt like my body had been run over by a freight train. I looked deathly ill for many days and had to go back on another fast to clear out the enormous dinner I had eaten in error. I survived, I suppose, so I could share my ignorance with you fourteen years later and save you the same mistake.

Before attempting any fasting or radical diet change, please check with your family doctor. The atmosphere in which you do a fast is important. No stress, meditate daily, no strenuous work-outs; it is a time to relax and renew the body.

Nutritional Breakdown of the Fasting Juice

Here is my simple survey of the basic foods that have become valuable allies to me, especially when I am tired from too much traveling, too many restaurant meals, or too many late work nights in general. My fasting juice recipe was developed over many years of experimenting, and has been a lifesaver for me on more than one occasion.

Garlic kills worms, helps to clear up skin problems, wards off coughs and colds, and lowers the blood pressure.

Recently the University of California at Irvine and Sloane Kettering Cancer Center in New York and Nutrition International in Irvine found that garlic extract retarded the growth of breast cancer cells by 50 percent, and that eating two or three medium cloves of garlic daily may reduce the risk of cancer (all types) by 10 to 100 percent. Kyolic or SGP can be purchased in health food stores and as aged garlic extracts, they are both odorless products.

If you include fresh garlic in your pre-fasting vegetable

juices, it will cleanse the blood. Garlic is a "natural antibiotic" containing sulfur, vitamins C, B_1, B_2, E, and K, calcium, copper, magnesium, potassium, phosphorous, selenium, zinc, and eighteen amino acids. It will help to remove any bacterial matter that is released from the intestinal tract into the blood stream, as it is a disinfectant and diuretic (ridding the body of excess water). This diuretic effect also acts to cleanse the cells and help the body eliminate excess fat.

By including raw garlic in your juice, you will eliminate the unpleasant toxin release reactions mentioned earlier. Once the garlic has purified your blood of toxic waste, your skin will cease to emit a garlic odor. It is important to refrain from strenuous exercise while fasting since exercise pushes the toxins into the muscles, causing pain and cramping.

Carrots are high in potassium, and beta carotene, which is converted into vitamin A by the body and stored in the liver. Carrots also contain vitamins B_1, B_2, B_6, four other B vitamins known as biotin, niacin (B_3), pantothenic acid (B_5) and folic acid. Calcium, copper, iron, magnesium, manganese, phosphorus, selenium, zinc, and eighteen amino acids are also found in carrots. Carrots are a good source of raw fiber, and help to lower cholesterol. It is possible to overdose on vitamin A because vitamin A is stored in the liver and is not "washed out" of the body through urination as are other vitamins. However, if you have symptoms of Vitamin A overdose, such as diarrhea, dry skin, itching of the skin, nausea, headaches, blurred vision, aching in the bones, and sore mouth and lips, a sufficient intake of vitamin C will help eliminate these toxic effects.[5] The vitamin B group is extremely complex because the "B's" all interact and some cannot be absorbed without the presence of another and too high a dose of one may wipe out another in the group. B vitamins are destroyed by the contraceptive pill, sulfur drugs,

---

5. Cited in Bob Flaws, *Cervical Dysplasia & Prostate Cancer* (Boulder, CO: Blue Poppy Press, 1990).

narcotics, estrogen pills, the caffeine in tea and coffee, alcohol, high doses of sugar and starch, vinegar, and laxatives. Raw egg white stops the absorption of biotin, so if you like to put raw eggs in health food drinks, be sure to separate the egg whites and include only the yolks in your drinks.

Celery is high in vitamins A and K, calcium, magnesium, and potassium. Celery also contains vitamins B_1, B_2, B_6, C, and E, copper, iron, manganese, phosphorous, selenium, zinc, and all amino acids. Celery is a diuretic and helps to lower blood pressure and clear away fatty deposits.

Tomatoes contain a type of carotene called lycopene, which has been shown to fight the growth of cancer cells. Tomatoes are high in vitamins A and C, and potassium. They also contain vitamins B_1, B_2, B_6, and E, biotin, niacin, pantothenic acid, folic acid, calcium, copper, iron, magnesium, manganese, phosphorous, selenium, zinc, and all amino acids.

Avocados are an excellent source of vitamins A, B_1, B_2, B_6, C, E, and K, niacin, pantothenic acid and folic acid, calcium, copper, iron, manganese, and zinc. Avocados are high in potassium, phosphorous, and magnesium, contain all the amino acids, and are rich in protein and fiber. Avocados also provide the unsaturated fats required for the absorption of vitamins A, D, E, and K, and are needed for the conversion process of carotene to vitamin A in the body. Unsaturated fats are essential for the growth of skin, nerves, blood, and arteries; they help break down and transport cholesterol, which is required by the brain, blood, nervous system, and liver. These fats assist adrenal, sex hormone, and bile production. Too little fat in a diet will lead to dry, wrinkled, scaly skin and blood cells that "stick together" and lack motility.

Parsley is more than just a garnish! It is high in vitamins A and C, potassium, and calcium. Parsley also contains vitamins B_1, B_2, B_6, E, and K, biotin, niacin, pantothenic acid and folic acid, copper, iron, magnesium, manganese, zinc, phosphorous, and three of the essential amino acids. Parsley, eaten raw, is also a breath freshener, and will remove onion or garlic tastes from the mouth.

Beets have the marvelous effect of cleaning out fat deposits from the liver, gallbladder, kidneys, adipose cells (where cellulite likes to gather), and blood cells. Beets stimulate the lymph system thanks to their chlorine content. Beets and beet tops (which can also be juiced) are high in potassium and vitamins A and K, and also contain vitamins B_1, B_2, B_6, C, and E, niacin, pantothenic acid, folic acid, calcium, copper, iron, magnesium, manganese, phosphorous, zinc, and all amino acids.[6]

Lemons offer quite a good supply of potassium, and vitamins C, K, and have small amounts of vitamins B_1, B_2, B_6, niacin, pantothenic acid, folic acid, calcium, copper, iron, magnesium, manganese, and phosphorous. They have an astringent effect on the blood for cleansing.

All of the above-mentioned juice ingredients contain natural salt, which is necessary for overall health and regulating the blood. Sodium combines with potassium to maintain the right water, alkaline, and acid balance in the tissues. Combining with the chlorine found in the beets, sodium helps to keep the lymph system in good order.

---

6. I actually use beets sparingly only when fasting, since they are on the eliminated foods list for kidney stones.

Afterword

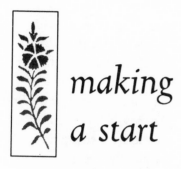

making
a start

THERE COMES A TIME IN OUR LIVES WHEN WE MUST, IF WE ARE ever to evolve, simply declare ourselves "healed." Twelve Step or Recovery Programs are powerful to get one on track, yet the final step of ceasing to speak about our wounds, our powerlessness and our victimhood has to happen if we are to move on to wholeness as complete individuals, able to stand alone without fear. There has to be a mental energy shift.

When I was involved in Recovery, or Un-covery actually—who needs to re-cover up anything—taking part in a Twelve-Step program for sexual abuse survivors, the fact that I had been abused seemed to come up in conversation with nearly every new person I met. They would talk about their childhood wounds. We swapped stories, we spoke "wound" and we bonded and felt safe in our wounded states of shared intimacy.

Then one day I decided that I had said "Hello, my name is Jeanne and I'm a sex abuse survivor" at one meeting too many. I think I even became bored with my own story; talking about it kept it alive and clouded living in the present. It happened, I survived, so be it. I didn't feel powerless. I was tired of saying that I was, it was negative reinforcement to my brain. I didn't feel that God or a Higher Power was outside of me, I knew I had been made in God's image and that the Divine also dwelt within me, and it was that part of me that had helped me survive in the first place. In realizing all those things, I could no longer comfortably go to another Survivor meeting, not if I was true to myself. For me to heal, somehow I had to do it without the meetings, to use the *principles* of the Steps in my daily life, by myself and, with the help of a therapist, do my own healing work to clear out the basic remnants of the past.

If I wanted to, I could complain about my abuse until I'm eighty years old. Yet what's the point? There is a great deal more that makes up "me," than my abuse. I'm also me getting on with my life, as best I can, making mistakes just like everyone else, and hopefully learning from them.

The decision to become a therapist, and my desire to help others, took me from my island shores to America, to the jungles of Mexico, and lead me to my husband—what he calls a "meaningful coincidence"—and with whose daily support, love, understanding, and occasional past transgression, has helped me become more and more of the woman I will be someday. I am forced to see my own issues through his. Meanwhile I help him look at his childhood wounds, and past and current behavior patterns.

No matter how far away I am from my husband our souls are always entwined. We bump each other up and along the higher path to greater spiritual understanding and ways of being through prayer, meditation and faith. Through our journey comes strength and clarity of purpose to face issues which must be dealt with for large or small breakthroughs and healings to occur. It is also easier to say, than to do.

Giving up compulsive behavior or addictions, whatever they are—pot, booze, cigarettes, pills, drugs, junk food, sugar, nail biting, nose picking, coffee, tea, binge eating, shopping, the telephone, drama and chaos, gambling, television, sex—is no day at the beach. They are all dependencies, barriers that keep the pain or the fear or the anger "down" inside where it is safe and we don't have to look at it. I am not being puritanical. God made me clean up my act bit by bit, kicking and screaming all the way.

No one can whine better than I can. No one can say the wrong thing at the wrong time, better than I can. Sometimes when the going got tough, I would think to myself: if I could drink without going into kidney failure I would; if I could take Valium without becoming a zombie I would; if I could smoke a Marlboro Light without blacking out, I would. And then I'd think, no I'd rather plod along facing everything I have to face without any form of "medication." Admitting the human frailties to myself somehow heals.

All systems of healing can be integrated into daily living—acupuncture and acupressure, herbal medicine, color therapy, Reiki Therapy, Network Chiropractic, Polarity Therapy, ear and nose piercing, gem therapy, aromatherapy, cleansing juice fasts. It is simply a matter of understanding how and why such systems are effective, many of them having served humanity most efficiently for thousands of years.

Healing takes time, but the sooner you understand the principles behind Oriental medicine, the sooner you will be on the road to freedom from ill-health. You will have a greater understanding of how your body actually functions.

As far as I am concerned, it all boils down to this: In order for the cycle of abuse and dis-ease to end—rather than to continue to affect generation after generation—women must heal themselves. When we heal, our families will have a better chance to heal too.

Remember the somewhat obvious fact: women become mothers by virtue of having children. Children come through us, never ours to possess, dogmatize or mistreat; they need to be loved, nurtured, protected, appreciated, listened to, encouraged, and praised. Be willing to listen with equal openness to the child you have brought into this world. Look at the awe and wonder and openness in your children's eyes and the clarity of the face. Remember that Jesus said that until you become as children you cannot enter the Kingdom of Heaven. The healing journey of the Self back to Innocence, a clean slate, a whole body, is available to us all.

We are living in a time when we must more and more assume responsibility for our bodies and our lives. Please feel free to contact me with your questions and your results. I pray that this work will serve you, and that you will share what you learn with others.

May God bless you and keep you safe from harm or ill-health.

Jeanne Elizabeth Blum
Woman Heal Thyself
Hiakulana
555 Hiaku Rd.
Haiku, Maui, HI 96708

a new view on five element theory

WHAT YOU ARE ABOUT TO READ IS NEW THOUGHT ON THE FIVE Element Theory. To the best of my knowledge, no one has examined the traditional Five Element chart from this perspective.

I have included this new thinking in *Woman Heal Thyself* purely to share with you information that may be of use as you delve deeper into Oriental medicine and begin to unravel the puzzle of your own medical history, perhaps some of it inherited. This way of looking at the Five Elements was of great help to me when I began to trace illness and the causes of death within my own family tree.

While I was relaxing, and reading a manuscript draft of *Woman Heal Thyself* for the first time, something caught my eye and I began to think in the following manner: if there were Five Elements, why were there only three generations of Grandparent, Parent and Child discussed in the traditional teachings of Five Element Theory? What about the other two elements? There should be corresponding generations for them as well.

It was clear to me that a Great Grandparent and Great-Great Grandparent level existed. The chart suddenly looked like an energetic format of incest and inbreeding for genetic study covering Five Generations in one family.

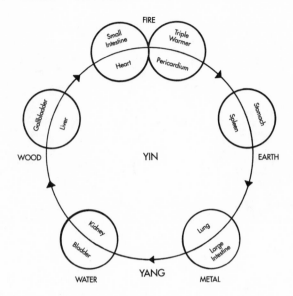

The Five Element chart showing the Yin organs and Yang organs.

What struck me as being even more amazing, is that the chart appears to suggest the ways emotional energetic imbalance and disease are passed from one generation to the next, and seems to indicate which sex carries a particular disease.

The Five Element Chart is neatly divided into a female side (the Yin inner organs) and a male side (the Yang outer organs). Because energetic imbalance manifests physically in the body, and is said to remain in "body memory," such imbalance could also be passed on genetically in the genes and chromosomes.

It occurred to me that the chart can be used to explain how diseases and addictions are passed from one generation to the next, or appear to skip a generation or two. I have attempted to demonstrate this through the Grandparent/Grandchild formulation by using what I call the Inner Flow Arrow Chart. The recessive gene is hidden in the Parent generation. Therefore, the body can be looked at in a physical, energetic, chemical, genetic, and algebraic manner.

The charts also appear to be a progression of meiosis or cell division. For example, diseases of the kidney are carried in the female inherited genes—X chromosome, the kidney being a Yin or female organ—that diseases of the stomach are carried in the male encoding and so forth. Diseases are genetically passed from Parent to Child, or from Grandparent to Grandchild. However, if a disease appears to be untraceable, the probability is that it originates in a generation that is further removed, and might be called, for convenience sake, a super-recessive gene or a super-super recessive gene, with the disease showing up in the great- or great-great-grandchild generation.

And then I wondered: If energetic emotional imbalance can be passed on through the genes, in the form of disease or addictions, creating the genetic personality through chromosome encoding, is it not possible for ancestor memory also to be transmitted with the emotions?

Should this prove to be the case and our ancestors' memories are found to survive in our genetic encoding, just like curly hair or blue eyes, could we simply access this memory load from time to time? Re-accessing their fears, their terrors, their experiences, their knowledge, which then become our nightmares or pleasing dreams while we sleep, or our visions while we wake, if the "trigger" situation is in place to reactivate or re-access these memories. The "trigger" just being like a password to enter a computer system. This would explain why for some people mathematics is so easy, or there are generations of gifted doctors in one family.

Scientists have told us we use only 10 percent of our brain. Is the other 90 percent perhaps a storage bank? And because we know that electrical exchange takes place within it, the brain can be said to be our own personal computer, running each individual "show" and that as a storage bank, all our ancestor memories are lodged in the brain cells, and when those cells are stimulated by daily living "triggers," they release their information to the conscious mind. As my husband would say "Where was an idea just before you had it?" Perhaps Plato said it best, "All knowledge is recollection."

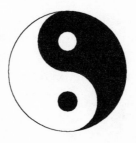

The traditional Yin Yang symbol

What about things that you just "know"—history, or medicine, or ancient people—yet you have never read about or been told about the subject? Or you have a familiar sense in a place you've never been, a feeling that you have indeed been there previously. A foreign country that feels like home, the moment you fly into its air space or step off a plane or train? From what source does that knowing come? Do you have a "green thumb" because your mother or grandmother did? But how did you get the plant knowledge she had and never discussed with you? Is the "collective unconscious" really inside our heads, that close to us if we somehow manage to access the information?

Is what we're dealing with here the seat of our intuitive, the birth place of "hunches," our "sixth sense"—the sense that is associated with no traditional organ—the sense that "knows" the future, is connected to God, and comes from the Divine Presence within us?

Some say the Soul, the all knowing, is located within the Pineal gland in the brain. Is that why we are now bound by the rule "brain dead" in terms of life support machinery when someone is ill or dying, so that we don't bury someone with a still live, electrically charged, thinking brain? Is that why so many ancient cultures insisted on cremation, for absolute release of the tangible thinking part of the Soul within the brain?

The traditional Yin-Yang symbol (the male within the female and the female within the male) can be looked at as a symbolic representation of the source of our being, on a cellular level. The symbol resembles a cell containing both DNA and

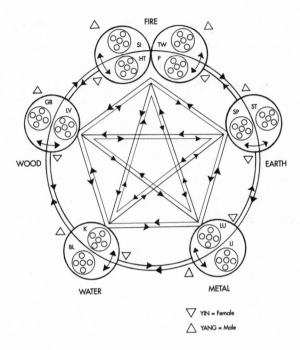

The complete flow of positive (Yang = △) and negative (Yin = ▽) energy throughout the human body from the Great-great-grandparent generation to Child.

RNA, the nucleic acid molecules that carry the genetic coding; DNA (deoxyribonucleic acid) carrying instructions for cellular processes while RNA (ribonucleic acid) transmits those instructions. Nucleic acid molecules, along with proteins, are the two ingredients essential for life on earth. The generational

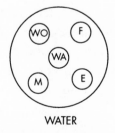

WATER

Five Elements "molecule."

father's genes are responsible for mixing the DNA. In the generational mother's genes, there is DNA which never mixes with that of the father's and is passed on without any changes to each female generation. It is the same with father to son DNA.

If all of the energetic exchanges within our body system were drawn into this traditional chart you would have a chart that looks like the chart on the page 291, right down to the cellular level.

Compare this Five Element Chart and the traditional genetic diagram for meiosis, or cell division. The circles within the circles also have the ability to divide yet again and again ad infinitum on an energetic basis, each unit exchanging energy according to the Five Element Theory, within each small individual element, there is another entire Five Element "world" with its own element at the center.

This orbiting "world" resembles a molecule with the nucleus at the center holding both the positive charge of the protons and the neutral charge of the neutrons, and the electrons with a negative charge, freely orbiting at different energetic levels.

People have talked and written about the theories of ancestor memory and the "collective unconscious" for many years. This chapter is about thinking: new thinking to stimulate you to ponder and ask questions about your family origins. Try to seek out relatives that are still alive, and compile as much family data as possible for future generations.

As a teenager, I knew there was something wrong with me. Perhaps four times a year I felt "hungry." Recently, I realized that I was genetically anorexic: traceable back to my maternal great-grandfather, who was fond of excesses in both food and sex. The women in my mother's family were all anorexic, bulimic, or both. Sex addiction afflicted the men. Stomach and Spleen were involved in each case. With my cousins of both sexes, the same great-grandfather passed on these disorders, to grandfather, to son. Maternally or paternally, women have eating problems and men have the sex addiction. It is a dominant, generational gene.

In 1994, I went on a five-day detoxing Large Intestine cleanse, drinking only fruit juices, psyllium husks, and colloidal bentonite with montmorillonite (clay). The result: hunger became a normal sensation, healing a genetic eating disorder by physically treating the "Child" organ—Large Intestine. Using the Parent Rule and detoxing cleanses, I am developing a method I believe will help cure genetic addictions and disorders.

In asking questions, we learn. We learn how to think, how to unleash the mind and set it free to solve problems and make life easier. The Forbidden Pregnancy Points System and this book came as the result of my posing one simple question to a kind and open teacher, Nancy Marchant. Her class was a safe place to explore, to heal, and to grow.

May this chapter serve you as you search for the secrets to staying healthy and living well.

Example: Earth Element

Here is the progression from Great-great-grandfather and Great-great-grandmother through Child generations in energetic flow of balance and low or excessive imbalance.

Earth is Great-great-grandparent of Fire

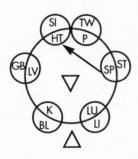

Spleen - - = Heart - -
Spleen + + = Heart + +

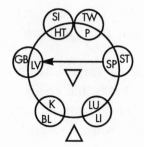

Earth is Great-grandparent of Wood

Spleen - = Liver - -
Spleen + = Liver + +

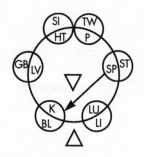

Earth is Grandparent of Water

Spleen   + = Kidney -
Spleen + + = Kidney -
Spleen - - = Kidney +

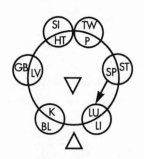

Earth is Parent of Metal

Spleen ≡ = Lung ≡
            (≡ balance)

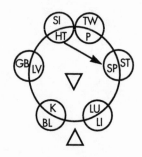

Earth is the Child of Fire

Spleen   = Heart
Spleen +   = Heart +
Spleen -   = Heart -
Spleen + + = Heart - -

 *the anti-miscarriage points*

When this book was first published I received many phone calls asking me for the anti-miscarriage points listed below. These points, mentioned in chapter 4, can also be used to stop abnormal uterine bleeding. I've also added points for edema.

ANTI-MISCARRIAGE:
    Spleen

	3	*Supreme White*
	10	*Sea of Blood*

    Large Intestine

	1	*Shang Yang or Extreme Yang*

    Bladder

	15	*Heart's Hollow (Shu)*
	17	*Diaphragm's Hollow (Shu)*
	18	*Liver's Hollow (Shu)*
	22	*Triple Burner's Hollow*
	23	*Kidney's Hollow (Shu)*
	31	*Upper Sacral Bone-Hole*
	32	*Second Sacral Bone-Hole*

ANTI-MISCARRIAGE (Cont.):
　Bladder (cont.)
　　　33　　　　　　　*Central Bone-Hole*
　　　34　　　　　　　*Lower Bone-Hole*
　Conception Vessel
　　　4　　　　　　　*First Gate*
　　　6　　　　　　　*Sea of Ch'i*
　Governing Vessel
　　　20　　　　　　　*One Hundred Convergences*

EDEMA:
　Spleen
　　　9　　　　　　　*Yin Mountain Spring*
　Liver
　　　3　　　　　　　*Great Surge*
　Conception Vessel
　　　5　　　　　　　*Stone Gate*
　　　7　　　　　　　*Yin Intersection*

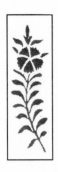

recommended reading

THE BOOKS LISTED HERE FALL INTO TWO CATEGORIES, THOSE I have read and those that come as recommended reading by different friends and colleagues.

Achterber, Jeanne. *Woman as Healer.* Boston: Shambhala, 1991

Amber, Rueben & A.M. Babey-Brooke. *Pulse Diagnosis: Detailed Interpretation for Eastern and Western Treatments.* Santa Fe, NM: Aurora Press, 1993

Arrien, Angeles, Ph.D. *The Four-Fold Way: Walking the Paths of the Warrior, Teacher, Healer, & Visionary.* San Francisco: Harper-Collins, 1993

Bauer, Cathryn. *Acupressure for Women.* Freedom, CA: Crossing Press, 1987

Bloomfield, Frena. *The Book of Chinese Beliefs.* New York: Avon Books, 1983

———. *Harmony Rules.* York Beach, ME: Samuel Weiser, 1987

Blum, Ralph H. *The Book of Runes.* New York: St. Martin's Press, 1982

——— and Susan Loughan, *The Healing Runes.* New York: St. Martin's Press, 1995

Bruyere, Rosalyn L. *Wheels of Light.* Sierra Madre, CA: The Crossing Press, 1989

Chaitow, Leon. *Candida Albicans*. Rochester, VT: Healing Arts Press, 1987

Chang, Jolan. *The Tao of Love and Sex*. New York: Penguin Books, 1977

Chia, Mantak. *Awaken Healing Energy Through the Tao*. Santa Fe, NM: Aurora Press, 1983

Chinen, Allan B. *Once Upon a Midlife*. Los Angeles, CA: Jeremy P. Tarcher, 1992

Cleary, Thomas. *The Immortal Sisters*. Boston: Shambhala, 1989

Connelly, Diane M. *Traditional Acupuncture: The Law of the Five Elements*. Columbia, MD: The Centre for Traditional Acupuncture, 1989

Dossey, Larry, M.D. *Healing Words: The Power of Prayer and the Practice of Medicine*. San Francisco: HarperCollins, 1993

Duerk, Judith. *Circle of Stones*. San Diego, CA: LuraMedia, 1989

Engel, Beverly. *The Emotionally Abused Woman*. New York: Ballantine Books, 1990

Estes, Clarissa Pinkola. *Women Who Run With the Wolves*. New York: Ballantine Books, 1992

Evans, Patricia. *The Verbally Abusive Relationship: How to Recognize It and How to Respond*. Expanded 2nd Edition. Holbrook, MA: Adams Media Corporation, 1996

Haas, Elson. *Staying Healthy With the Seasons*. Berkeley, CA: Celestial Arts, 1981

Harary, Keith and Weintraub, Pamela. *Inner Sex in 30 Days*. New York: St. Martin's Press, 1990

Hay, Louise. *You Can Heal Your Life*. Carson, CA: Hay House, 1987

Hodgkinson, Neville. *Will to Be Well: The Real Alternative Medicine*. York Beach, ME: Samuel Weiser, 1986

Hendricks, Gay and Kathlyn. *Conscious Loving*. New York: Bantam Books, 1992

Jacobowitz, Ruth, S. *150 Most-Asked Questions About Mid-life, Sex, Love & Intimacy*. NY: William Morrow/Hearst, 1993

Kavanaugh, Philip. *Magnificent Addiction.* Lower Lake, CA: Aslan Publishing, 1992

Lee, John. *The Flying Boy: Healing the Wounded Man.* Austin, TX: New Man's Press, 1987

——*Recovery Plain and Simple: Co-dependency and Adult Children.* Deerfield Beach, FL: Health Communication, 1990

Leonard, Linda Schierse. *On the Way to the Wedding.* Boston: Shambhala, 1986

——. *The Wounded Woman.* Boston: Shambhala, 1982

McCarthy, Barry and Emily. *Intimate Marriage.* New York: Carroll & Graf Publishers, 1992

Millman, Dan. *Sacred Journey of the Peaceful Warrior.* Tiburon, CA: HJ Kramer Inc., 1991

Murdoch, Maureen. *The Heroine's Journey.* Boston: Shambhala, 1990

Northrup, Christiane, M.D. *Women's Bodies, Women's Wisdom.* New York: Bantam Books, 1994

Scarf, Maggie. *Intimate Partners.* New York: Ballantine Books, 1987

Shealy, Norman C., and Caroline M. Myss. *The Creation of Health: The Emotional, Psychological, and Spiritual Responses That Promote Health.* Rev. ed. Walpole, NH: Stillpoint Publishing, 1993

——The Shealy Institute, 1328 East Evergreen, Springfield, MO 65803

Sheehy, Gail. *The Silent Passage.* New York: Random House, 1992

Stein, Diane. *A Woman's Book of Healing.* St. Paul, MN: Llewellyn, 1987

Tannen, Deborah. *You Just Don't Understand.* New York: Ballantine Books, 1990

Teeguarden, Iona Marsaa. *Acupressure Way of Health.* Berkeley, CA: University of California Press, 1966

Veith, trans. *The Yellow Emperor's Classic of Internal Medicine.* Berkeley, CA: University of California Press, 1966

Walters, J. Donald (Kriyananda). *How to Spiritualize Your Marriage.* Nevada City, CA: Crystal Clarity Publishers, 1991

Weed, Susun S. *Wise Woman Herbal for the Childbearing Year.* Woodstock, New York: Ash Tree Publishing, 1985

Weiss, Brian L. *Through Time Into Healing.* New York: Simon & Schuster, 1992

Welwood, John. *Journey of the Heart.* New York: HarperCollins, 1990

Wilhelm, Richard. *The I Ching or Book of Changes.* New Jersey: Princeton University Press, 1990

Wing, R.L. *The Tao of Power.* New York: Doubleday, 1986

Woodman, Marion. *Addiction to Perfection.* Toronto, Canada: Inner City Books, 1982

Woodman, Marion. *The Pregnant Virgin.* Toronto, Canada: Inner City Books, 1985

Woodman, Marion. *The Ravaged Bridegroom.* Toronto, Canada: Inner City Books, 1990

Zimmerman, Jack and Coyle, Virginia. *The Practice of Council.* Ojai, CA: Ojai Foundation, 1990

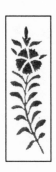

index

ALSO REFER TO "Diagnostic Reference for Ailments A-Z" on pages 205 through 230 for an alphabetical listing of specific common ailments.

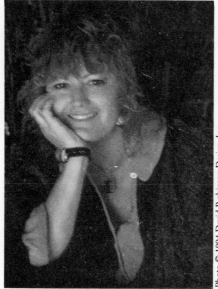

JEANNE ELIZABETH BLUM was born in Bermuda and has lived all over the world. In 1989, she founded the Healing Light Therapies Centre in Bermuda. She holds degrees in Massage Therapy and Oriental Massage Therapy from the San Francisco School of Massage and the Heartwood Institute in northern California. She has studied Swedish Esalen Massage and Jin Shin Do Acupressure and Auricular Therapy. She has trained with Norman Shealy, M.D., a neurosurgeon at Duke and the founder of both the American Holistic Medical Association and the Pain Rehabilitation Center at the Shealy Institute in Missouri. She is a practitioner of acupressure and auricular therapy, and treats clients suffering from addiction, emotional imbalance, and physical ailments.